Yoga Mastery: Navigating the Art and Business of Teaching

Strategies for Yoga Professionals to Cultivate a Satisfying Career Path

Copyright © 2023

All Rights reserved. This book may not be reproduced in whole or in part, stored in a retrieval system, or transmitted in any form or by any means — electronic, mechanical, or other — without written permission from the publisher, except by a reviewer, who may quote brief passages in a review.

The material in this book is intended for educational purposes only. No expressed or implied guarantee of the effects of the use of the recommendations can be given or liability taken.

Contents

Introduction

Part I: Becoming a Yoga Teacher

Chapter 1: Teaching Today
Chapter 2: Presenting Yourself as a Teacher

Part II: Getting Down to Business

Chapter 3: Yoga Business Basics
Chapter 4: Building Your Business
Chapter 5: Marketing Your Business
Chapter 6: Social Media
Chapter 7: Forming Good Professional Relationships
Chapter 8: Managing Your Business Finances

Part III: Teaching Well

Chapter 9: Class Planning and Preparation
Chapter 10: Teaching a Class
Chapter 11: Self-Care

Conclusion: Light Up the World
Index

Introduction: The narrator, a passionate yoga practitioner since his teenage years, becomes a yoga teacher after eleven years of rigorous asana practice. Initially feeling too young and unqualified, he enrolls in a teacher training course under the guidance of Cyndi Lee. This experience motivates him to become a teacher. After the training, he joins a community of like-minded yogis, desiring to live in harmony with nature and mindful of their choices. Teaching yoga was uncommon at the time, but the narrator perseveres, and by 1998, with the growing popularity of yoga, he transitions from a fledgling teacher to a sought-after one. However, commercialization brings challenges, with debates about diluting ancient yoga ideas and the elitist perception due to celebrity adoption. In 2010, the narrator meets Taro Smith, and together they develop an online course for yoga teachers, addressing the challenges of teaching yoga in a crowded market. With the success of the course, they establish their company, 90 Monkeys, dedicated to providing online and in-person educational resources for yoga teachers.

Part I

BECOMING A YOGA TEACHER

CHAPTER ONE

Teaching Today

Millions of people have experienced yoga's benefits. Some have found that it lessens pain or stress, and some have incorporated yoga into their meditation or spiritual practice. Many others find that yoga just *feels* good and increases their overall sense of well-being.

Yoga has traditionally been seen as a path to heightened consciousness and mindfulness, though this aspect is increasingly less emphasized in the West. The practice facilitates a profound awareness of how body, mind, and spirit are linked and how each individual is connected to all life on the planet.

In a world dominated by nonstop activity and the proliferation of high-tech devices, yoga is one of the few popular endeavors that require only a sticky mat and a commitment to practice. No technology is needed.

As a yoga practitioner, you know that yoga practice is sometimes the only time of day when someone truly unplugs, enters a state of calm, moves their body, and simply breathes. As a yoga teacher, you have the honor and privilege of guiding people through that process — a process that is sometimes delightful and often challenging, but always rewarding.

Teaching yoga is often thought of as a lifestyle business. This means that you have chosen a pastime that is central to your own lifestyle and are taking the chance that you can create a career, or supplement other income, by devoting yourself to it.

We are called to teach because we love any excuse to get on our yoga mats, cherish watching our students develop, and likely have a pronounced aversion to cubicle life, endless meetings, and uncomfortable shoes!

The Good News about Teaching Yoga Today

Yoga Journal and Yoga Alliance, the professional organization representing yoga teachers, studios, and schools, conducted an extensive study into the current state of yoga in the United States.* According to their 2016 "Yoga in America" report, 36.7 million people practice yoga, up from 20.4 million in 2012. Yoga is not only growing, it's booming. In fact, 28 percent of all Americans have taken a yoga class at some point in their lives. More men and more older people are practicing than ever before: in 2015, there were approximately 10 million male practitioners and almost 14 million practitioners over the age of fifty.

Yogis are also contributing to the economy, spending over $16 billion annually on classes, yoga clothing, equipment, and accessories, up from $10 billion in 2012. Evidently, yoga is enticing: 34 percent of Americans say they are somewhat likely or very likely to practice yoga in the next twelve months — which is equal to more than 80 million Americans. Why do they want to try yoga? They reported wanting to increase their flexibility, relieve stress, and improve their fitness levels.

According to the survey, yoga is an increasing part of life in the United States. Since 2012, the percentage of Americans aware of yoga has jumped from 75 percent to 90 percent. One in three Americans have tried yoga on their own (not in a class) at least once.

The findings also indicate that yoga practitioners tend to have a positive self-image: they are 20 percent more likely than nonpractitioners to report that they have "good balance," "good physical agility or dexterity," or "good range of motion or flexibility" or that they "give back to the community."

The study also shows that yoga students are highly concerned about their health, their community, and the environment. More than 50 percent of practitioners report trying to eat sustainable foods and live green, compared with about a third of the general population. Nearly half of yoga practitioners report donating time to their communities, compared with just 26 percent of those who don't practice yoga.

Perhaps not surprisingly, yoga teachers and teacher trainees are even more tuned in to environmental and social issues and to living and eating consciously than other yoga practitioners: 22 percent of yoga teachers and trainees are vegetarians, compared with 8 percent of other yoga practitioners and 3 percent of the general public; and 60 percent of yoga teachers and trainees use natural health and beauty products, compared with 44 percent of other yoga practitioners and 21 percent of the general public.

Statistics like these support what has always been true in the yoga circles in which I run: yogis are living life with more self-awareness and positive self-regard, and as a result of this increased sensitivity, they are making an encouraging difference for the environment and in their communities.

What does all this mean for you as a teacher or aspiring teacher? The demand for yoga teachers is higher than ever — and unlikely to decrease anytime soon.

The Challenges of Being a Yoga Teacher

With statistics like those above, it's clear that as a yoga teacher, you're part of a movement that is growing exponentially and one that is becoming more and more a part of life in our society. As exciting as this can be, it's important to recognize that there are also challenges that come along with becoming or being a teacher. This book will help you understand and minimize these challenges, see how they apply to your specific situation, and find ways to manage them with skill and finesse.

First, with the growing popularity of yoga, the demand for teacher training has created a small army of yoga teachers all over the world, and you are just one of them. It's not as easy to stand out as it used to be.

At the same time, because of this popularity, modern yoga is sometimes criticized as being overly commercialized. Awareness of these criticisms can make it difficult to feel confident promoting yourself, spreading the word about your teaching, or asking to be compensated for your time and energy.

What's more, even though you have probably invested lots of time and money in developing your yoga education, teaching yoga has not traditionally been a lucrative career.

Yoga and Money

The ethical aspects of combining yoga with business, money, and marketing can be troubling: 50 percent of yoga teachers polled in our courses reported feeling awkward about charging for their teaching. But a great many of these teachers reported that they felt uncomfortable because of what *other* people think about yoga and money.

The reality is that yoga means different things to different people. Here are three common categories or belief systems:

1. Those who think that yoga should maintain its roots solely in an esoteric and spiritual practice and are therefore more likely to have a hard time with the commercial side of yoga and its marketing and promotion.
2. Those who see yoga teaching as a hobby or side job. These yogis are usually fortunate enough to be able to teach without worrying about compensation.
3. Those who live fully in the twenty-first-century, modern world and see teaching yoga as a profession through which they earn a living.

If you're serious about teaching yoga as an occupation, I'd like to help you understand why the third category is the clear choice and how the other two belief systems can confuse the profession of teaching yoga.

SHOULD YOGA BE FREE?

Every time a teacher offers a yoga class for free (or teaches for very little) they are *paying* to teach that class. They bought the gas for their car to get there, they paid for parking outside the studio, and potentially they rented the space too. In other words, they spent more money than they earned. Whenever a class is given away, that choice influences the market, thereby undermining others who depend on their teaching income to support themselves. I almost never teach for free, and when I do it's typically for a benefit in which participants have donated to the cause. It's fine to teach for free once in a while, but be mindful not to make this your modus operandi.

Yoga is now a $16 billion industry in the United States. Marketing of yoga accessories — everything from mats, props, and bags to yoga-specific clothing and even jewelry and nutritional supplements — has exploded. Promoters organize yoga conferences and festivals with lots of tangentially related activities, such as music concerts, slacklining, hula hooping, stand-up paddle boarding, and even wine tasting. With the promotional efforts that accompany these enterprises, criticism is inevitable.

For yoga teachers thinking of yoga as both a practice and a profession, it's helpful to understand the current state of affairs, and also to know a little of the history of yoga in both India and the West. Yoga practice and teaching in the West have been heavily influenced by particular schools of yoga with a focus on spiritual enlightenment — the traditions of Patanjali's classical yoga and Advaita Vedanta — using yoga to transcend our identification with the material world. Practitioners of these forms of yoga renounced material wealth and other forms of indulgence, many taking vows of celibacy. But these schools of yoga and their philosophies are not the only ones; they just happen to be the forms that gained an early foothold in the West. As a result, the yoga world is dealing with the residual effects of this one outlook.

MONEY AND YOGA IN THE DISTANT PAST

Once upon a more patriarchal time, thousands of years ago in India, the teacher-student relationship was focused on *dakshina* (the sacred compensation or sacrifice), rooted in the notion that the student, in complete deference to the teacher, would pay whatever fee the teacher demanded. The demand was not always explicit, just assumed. The patriarchal model was guru above, student below.

In the West, education and the teacher-student relationship are based more on parity than on hierarchy or authority. For yoga in the

West, and yoga in the twenty-first century, a new paradigm is required.

Those who object to treating yoga as a business perhaps fail to consider that yoga is not solely a spiritual practice: it is a form of education, encompassing physical activity, wellness, philosophy, and even history. And if yoga is a multifaceted form of education rather than an esoteric spiritual quest, it stands to reason that, as with other forms of training, such as piano lessons or a language course, a yoga education costs money. It is time for a more modern paradigm in the West, one that regards teaching yoga, like other forms of schooling, as a legitimate profession.

While sleazy marketing is unattractive in any field, and particularly in yoga, yoga cannot be kept free of promotion or commerce. If yoga teachers do not promote the merits of yoga and their own expertise in teaching it, then how will people find the path to those benefits? The great rewards of yoga are worth sharing with the world. The distinctive gifts that yoga teachers can offer their students are worth publicizing, and in our modern world they have monetary value.

It might help to apply some fundamental yoga philosophy to the controversy. *The Yoga Sutras of Patanjali* (second century CE) discusses two concepts for explaining reality: *prakriti* and *purusha*.

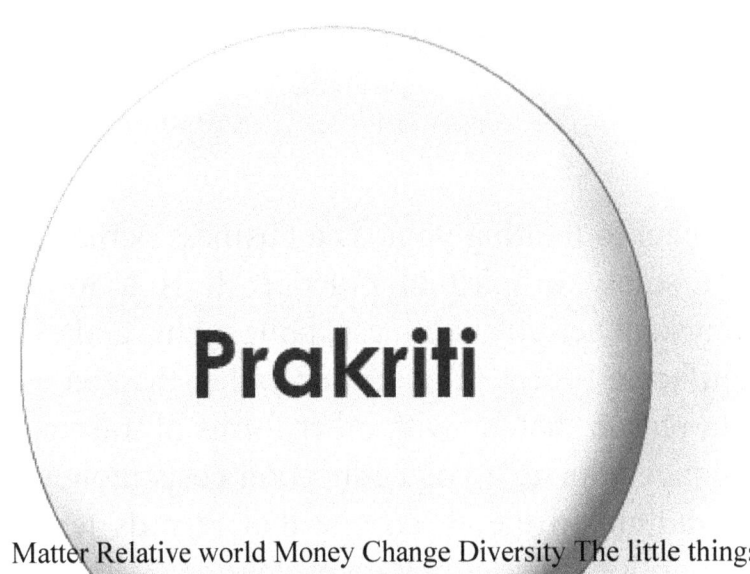

Matter Relative world Money Change Diversity The little things

Spirit The absolute The eternal Permanence Oneness The big picture

Prakriti encompasses matter, the material world, feelings and emotions, anything that changes, diversity, and the "little things," including money. *Purusha* encompasses spirit, the absolute, the eternal, that which does not change.

Purusha-prioritizing traditions see the material world as a problem to be fixed or to withdraw from. Sayings such as "I am not this body, I am not this mind" and "All of that is an illusion" come from a school identified with *purusha*. Strict followers attempt to suppress their feelings, stanch desire, conquer the human ego, and retreat from the real world through meditation in order to attain the beautiful vision of *purusha*. An exclusive focus on other-than-the-world makes it difficult to negotiate our twenty-first-century sphere.

There is an alternative view that embraces both *prakriti* and *purusha*. It is embodied in the Tantric schools of yoga, which are not as well known in the West. Tantra has come to be thought of as all about sexuality, but it is actually a much broader body of yoga and philosophy, one that addresses all aspects of human life. (To learn more about the origins of Tantra, we recommend *The Origins of Yoga and Tantra* by Geoffrey Samuel or *The Alchemical Body* by David G. White.)

Embracing both *prakriti* and *purusha* allows us to acknowledge that there are mouths to feed, worthy organizations working to make a difference that need our support, bills to pay, and kids to put through college. None of this is illusory; it is real.

Dichotomies that characterize yoga as beautiful and consumerism as ugly are neither helpful nor realistic. In fact, there is no escaping consumerism through yoga; humans, like everything else in the food chain, must eat and consume resources. The more interesting and important question is, How can we create a paradigm for thinking about money and consumerism that is ethical, conscious, and sustainable?

The Vicious Cycle of Yoga Teaching

I started the "90 Minutes" course because I knew what a privilege it is to teach yoga and live the lifestyle of a yogi. However, as a trainer of yoga teachers and a teacher myself, I was witnessing firsthand the struggles we went through to make ends meet. Over and over I saw teachers in what I came to call the "vicious cycle of yoga teaching." It goes like this:

1. Run all over town teaching eighteen or more classes a week to make ends meet.
2. Oops, no time for your own practice! No time to plan classes!
3. Teach subpar class because of lack of practice, inspiration, or groundedness.
4. Get home, have no time for reflection, fun, recreation, or family.

5. Get up the next day with even less inspiration, and teach to a dwindling number of students.
6. Make insufficient money to pay bills, afford necessary continuing education, or have much-needed free time.
7. Repeat.

Seeing good teachers teaching too many classes per week in order to pay bills and with no time or money for continuing education is painful. Many injure themselves during demonstrations because they have not been able to give time to their own practice and therefore stay strong in their bodies. Their classes and students inevitably suffer as a result.

Witnessing the graduates of my teacher trainings struggling to such a severe degree led me to put as much time into studying business as I had put into studying yoga philosophy. I wanted to help other yoga teachers, and by extension their students, by teaching them professional business practices.

Studying business and marketing gave me valuable tools, and it also taught me that there are two realities you need to face as a yoga teacher. Here they are, along with my suggestions for navigating them:

1. Most American full-time yoga teachers fall into the vicious cycle, especially new ones. Some teachers manage to avoid it, but given the changing nature of the market, there's no guarantee that you will be able to. I suggest that you keep this reality in mind and try to avoid falling into the cycle to the best of your ability, by not teaching more classes than you can happily handle (see pages 72–78) and by building your own practice time into your schedule every week.
2. We cannot control the market because there will always be yoga teachers willing to work for very little — since either they are new and eager to work or they are treating their teaching as a hobby. The choice to teach for less than market value unfortunately devalues the services all yoga professionals offer, so ultimately we must make the best of what the market will bear. The good news is that the more educated you are about professional business practices, the more likely it is that the market will reward you.

Your practice, your teaching, and your classes all benefit from your ability to view yoga as a valuable profession in today's world. Your students need you to be as skillful at life's practicalities as you are on the mat. As I hope is now clear, yoga and everyday life actually can't be separated.

TEACHER TRAINING

In addition to being able to teach a sequence of poses, yoga teachers would be wise to have an education in yoga alignment, therapeutic application, and the rich history and philosophy of yoga. Typically, based on Yoga Alliance standards, two hundred hours is the minimum adequate training time, with five hundred hours being the pinnacle of training. In some ways these numbers are arbitrary. Teaching yoga, like the practice of yoga, is a lifelong endeavor, and as such, continuing education and being a student for the long haul are essential to teaching yoga well.

Training programs vary from trainer to trainer and from school to school. Furthermore, some styles of yoga emphasize alignment, form, and philosophy more than others do.

You need a teacher trainer who has been well trained herself. Ask your teacher or program coordinator the following questions:

- Are you a graduate of a two-hundred-hour or five-hundred-hour training?
- Are you a graduate of more than one teacher training program?
- Did the style of yoga you trained in emphasize alignment and form? Philosophy?
- Who are your teachers? Are your trainers known for working with students on form, alignment, and injury prevention during the practice?
- Do you have any other credentials, such as being a licensed physical therapist or massage therapist or having a sports medicine background?

The Full Scope of Teaching Yoga Today

Yoga classes are often a refuge for students, a rare and precious place of quiet, reflection, and connection with self and with community. The spaces where we teach can often feel sacred, places where something special happens. But we aren't preachers or gurus. We don't tell others what to believe.

What we do is teach asana, a physical practice, informed by years of tradition and philosophy. We are in the business of offering a path to spiritual health and wellness. The multifaceted nature of our endeavor (art and profession, involving body, mind, and spirit) may strike some as paradoxical, but this multifaceted, twenty-first-century educational paradigm is empowering. Embrace it.

---

* The full study results are available at
www.yogaalliance.org/Portals/0/2016%20Yoga%20in%20America%20Study%20RESULTS.pdf.

CHAPTER TWO

Presenting Yourself as a Teacher

Longtime yogis are accustomed to self-awareness, self-inquiry, and self-assessment. These skills are also vitally important to yoga teachers. Yes, we must understand our students' expectations and motivations (and we'll discuss how to do that), but we can't thrive without understanding our own expectations and motivations or without having a clear awareness of our strengths and weaknesses.

I suggest you assess yourself in three categories: skilled yoga teacher, exemplary yoga teacher, and successful yoga teacher. This process will reveal your assets and deficiencies, as well as the actions you can take to improve. It will also help you develop a fuller and richer understanding of exactly why and how you teach.

What do I mean by *skilled, exemplary,* and *successful*? Here's how I define these terms for yoga teachers:

Skilled: Skilled at teaching, competent
Exemplary: Able to serve as a role model and example for others
Successful: Fulfilling personal career goals

This is not a progression. I don't mean that you should first work toward being skilled and then, once you've achieved that, move on to becoming exemplary. And, to be clear, I'm not suggesting that success will inevitably follow from being skilled and exemplary. What's more, none of these objectives is necessarily better than the others. The most skilled teachers may not be the best role models. Wonderful role models may not be the most successful teachers. You could reach your own personal career goals with gaps in your skills.

What I mean is that you should strive to attain a balance among all these objectives. When someone asks if you are a skilled teacher, an exemplary one, or a successful one, it is possible to say, "All of the above!"

Let's examine each category more closely.

The Skilled Yoga Teacher

A skilled yoga teacher is one who knows his stuff. He has been well trained and mentored by an experienced teacher, strives to remain current, and maintains a regular practice of his own. Because he understands alignment, he can offer good adjustments, both verbal and physical. His competence allows him to embody what he is teaching.

Skilled teachers offer a balance in the amount of instruction they offer — not too much, nor too little, but just enough. They understand the importance of silence. They prepare for their classes and observe their students well enough to teach the students who are actually in the room, even if this means altering their prepared class plan.

Skilled teachers produce good results because they meet students where they are, while also inspiring joyful perseverance. They look for and acknowledge progress rather than perfection. And they offer the kind of verbal cues and demonstrations that allow students to experience tangible shifts in their bodies.

Finally, a skilled teacher manages class time well. She begins and ends on time and balances the amount of time spent holding on the left and right sides, and on practicing standing poses and inversions, for example. (Teachers are not inherently better than students at managing time, so watch the clock or use a stopwatch in your preparations if necessary.)

The Not-So-Skilled Teacher

To get crystal clear about what makes a skilled teacher, it can be helpful to look at a few counterexamples. One flaw is expecting a student to be someone they are not or inflating a student's expectations beyond safe levels. Or a teacher might have insightful things to say but deliver them in a boring monotone. Unskilled teachers might also make students feel inferior, small, or talked down to. An unskilled teacher might make grandiose claims, like the ability to diagnose and cure a student's ailment. Worse yet, an unskilled teacher might convey the attitude that it's "my way or the highway."

The Exemplary Yoga Teacher

I define this type of teacher as a role model and example for others. He is both inspirational and down-to-earth. He has boundaries but is also available. He is authentic and so encourages students to be themselves as well. He follows a code of ethics that helps him move in the world with sensitivity and consideration for others and a high regard for the teacher-student relationship (see more on yoga teacher ethics in the section below). This teacher embraces collaboration with colleagues and is community oriented. With students and colleagues, and in the larger community, he embodies warmth and caring.

Despite these almost saintly qualities, an exemplary teacher is relentlessly real — honest, trustworthy, and fair. (This teacher understands that he is being paid and so wants his students to get extra value for their money.) While some students may want to place this teacher on a pedestal and view him as somehow superhuman, the teacher does not allow it. (Exemplary teachers want to be on mats, not on pedestals!) Without being falsely self-deprecating, an exemplary teacher acknowledges her own foibles. While confident in her role as teacher, she is also always learning and sometimes struggling. It's not a weakness to acknowledge difficulty; in fact, it can be a bridge to greater connection.

Modern Ethics: Beyond the Yamas *and* Niyamas

Almost every yoga teacher training program has a section on ethics, specifically the *yamas* and *niyamas* as outlined in Patanjali's *Yoga Sutras*. Ethics are particularly important in the teacher-student relationship in yoga because students may be vulnerable when they come to us for practice. It's vital that we instill their trust in us as professionals. A natural power differential is inherent in the teacher-student relationship. Therefore, we teachers need to be extra accountable as role models and hold ourselves to high standards. To read more about conduct and ethics pertaining to the teacher-student relationship, Google the "California Yoga Teachers Association Code of Conduct," which was written by veteran teacher Judith Hanson Lasater in 1995.

The *yamas* and *niyamas*, the first and second limbs of Patanjali's eight limbs of yoga, are the pragmatic principles and "rules" that were created to guide people's actions given the karmic, or cause-and-effect, nature of the world. In that karmic world we need human decency and accountability.

But karma isn't the whole picture. Its opposite is known as *lila. Lila* encompasses divine play, vulnerability, ambiguity, and the fact that anything can happen. As humans we are vulnerable to what the world dishes out, and the future is uncertain and unpredictable.

The *yamas* and *niyamas* are important and straightforward, and yet they don't quite account for a world that is also *lilic*. In one moment your life could be calm, and in the next breath it could change forever if a family member is hit by a car, your spouse gets laid off, or your health takes a turn for the worse.

Don't get me wrong — the *yamas* and *niyamas* are essential, and I wouldn't want to live in the world without them. Yet it's important to recognize that they originated as part of an ascetical paradigm meant to encourage seekers to move away from the world of social contracts.

Most third graders have been taught the equivalent of the *yamas* and *niyamas* ("don't steal," "give credit where it is due," "don't lie," "be clean," etc.) and learned to follow them. As yoga teachers we are ready for more. It is time to take ethics one step further and into modern times. We can do this by recognizing that we live in a world that is both karmic (predictable) and *lilic* (unpredictable). To put it plainly, having modern ethics means having your "ducks in a row" or having your act together. It means creating basic stability in your life so that when *lila* happens you can roll with the play of the universe rather than getting run over by it. Being prepared for any possibility means that you can create opportunities out of challenges rather than being a victim to them.

Why is this approach more ethical? Because when your life falls apart and you're not prepared, your problems inevitably become other people's problems. Take, for example, the yoga teacher who kept putting off getting health insurance until one day she was diagnosed with a serious health issue requiring extensive surgery. To cover her medical bills, the community had to rally to put together benefit classes and raise funds on her behalf. Or the person who put off getting snow tires on his car and then got stuck in the snow, blocking a family's driveway. Now he not only had let his coworkers down because he couldn't get to work but also impacted the four people in the house, who were now unable to get on with their day! Examples like these are endless.

Another thing to consider is this: if the *yamas* and *niyamas* are part of a yoga teacher's curriculum, why do we see so many yoga teachers breaking ethical contracts and lacking professional responsibility?

Herein lies the problem. If ethics exist only in a karmic world that yogis are aiming to escape from, then they can easily blame their "elevated state" as the reason for their violating ethical standards. In short, the guru gets a pass. A teacher who blames her transgressions or lack of responsibility on her spirituality is doing what is called "spiritual bypassing."

Modern, professional, and ethical teachers are, in Sanskrit, *auchitya*: "filled with appropriateness." They demonstrate awareness and understand the world they live in. In summary, these teachers:

- understand the features of a social contract (*yamas* and *niyamas*) and know that they are not exempt from its precepts.
- are functional and stable in their embodied life. How? By inviting vulnerability (*lila*) rather than being victimized by it.
- can embrace the paradox of social contract (karma) and divine play (*lila*).
- have their act together!

The more of an authority you are in your field, and the more privileges you receive because of that authority, the more accountable and responsible you have to be. The best leaders surround themselves with a system of checks and balances — or a high council to advise them on decisions and to call them out when they're buying into their own hype. These leaders are able to take feedback well and openly seek guidance from others.

Take some time to think about your life and how you can increase stability and harness a system of checks and balances. Some ideas include hiring a therapist, putting a studio manager in place, seeking the support of a mentor or friends who can be frank with you, having an attorney you can call upon on short notice, assembling a business team, having godparents for your children, setting up retirement and contingency funds, having life insurance, staying on top of car maintenance, seeking help from family, having a list of pet sitters you can call on, and lining up a team of health professionals for you and your family.

A Word on Charisma

While an exemplary teacher is humble, she also has a presence. Some would call this charisma. Although charisma might seem like a quality you have to be born with, everyone has a spark inside. It's just a matter of uncovering your light and letting it shine.

Martha Beck wrote a fantastic article on her belief that everyone (wallflowers included) has an innate and intangible "It" factor. As an example, she used the celebrity beagle Uno, the first of his breed to win the prestigious Westminster Kennel Club Dog Show in 2008 (see www.oprah.com/spirit/Charisma-and-Self-Confidence-Martha-Becks-Strategy). In her article Beck points out that despite being a beagle, often considered less interesting than more exotic breeds, this particular dog charmed the crowd and won the show with a standing ovation. She described how Uno shone his attention on everyone around him and how he exuded confidence, owned the ring, and held an elegant posture with ease.

There are many ways to unveil your natural charisma. Simple steps include making eye contact, standing and sitting up straight, speaking a bit more quickly, and mirroring the other person's body language when you're in conversation. However, having charisma mostly comes from "owning" your own space while turning your attention toward others. People pay attention to the person who is paying attention to them!

Having charisma is not inauthentic. It isn't an attempt to dazzle or garner adoration. Instead it is motivated by the teacher's genuine desire to optimize her ability to educate and be of service. It's a way of connecting.

The Not-So-Exemplary Teacher

A not-so-exemplary teacher may be talented and have much to offer as a role model but may hold himself back and get in his own way, meaning that instead of trusting himself, he is mired in self-doubt or negative self-talk.

Unfortunately, not all yoga teachers are well prepared to serve and give value to students. In some cases, a teacher tries too hard to make a good impression and then ends up coming across as inauthentic. Some teachers act deceptively inside the yoga studio to live up to the yogi image they have created but have a completely different personality outside the studio. Another limitation in a not-so-exemplary teacher is neglecting to listen to or understand her students.

The Successful Yoga Teacher

Everyone has a different definition of success. For our purposes here, I would define a successful yoga teacher as one who is bringing in a consistent and healthy income, is teaching the kind of students she enjoys working with, and has her desired schedule of private lessons and a well-attended schedule of group classes. A successful teacher may also be well known and respected in her community.

I see success as stemming from two different categories of personal qualities: those that are deep and reflective, and those that are superficial.

Deep Aspects of Successful Teachers

Deep aspects of success arise from conscious thought about what kind of success we want. One teacher's definition of success may be quite different from that of other teachers or of the yoga world at large.

A teacher who is successful on her own terms takes into account how much money she wishes and needs to make and how many students and what types of student she wants to work with. She knows her core values and why she has made these choices. Her thinking about these questions helps her formulate a clear mission statement (which we'll discuss on pages 35–36). In addition to knowing what kind of success you want, to be successful you'll also have to take actions and develop habits to make your vision into a reality. Overall, success requires goals, vision, and discipline.

BEING TRUE TO YOURSELF

As yoga has become more popular, trends and fads have proliferated — hot flow, yoga with themed and DJed music, glow-in-the-dark yoga, and so forth. It's not unusual to see hybrid offerings that combine yoga and wine tasting, yoga and chocolate, or yoga and pole dancing! Once you have defined your values and goals, you may choose to explore this sort of innovation in your teaching. And if you prefer to maintain a more traditional path, you can do so gracefully and professionally, without feeling threatened and without condemning or mocking those who do otherwise.

Superficial Qualities of Successful Teachers

There are certain other qualities that may contribute to success that I call superficial because we don't have to dig deep to attain them: we were born with them or came by them earlier in life. Some of these qualities include a certain mystique, something about an instructor's personality that seems to create an atmosphere in the classroom that makes students want to come back.

- *Beauty:* A teacher who is attractive or good-looking by society's standards, or a former model or actor trained in effective self-presentation, may have a greater chance of success. Of course we hope this teacher is also skilled and exemplary, but sadly, in this world people often choose eye candy over competence and character.
- *Connections:* Any teacher who has good professional connections to begin with will naturally have a career advantage.
- *Timing:* Being in the right place at the right time can help. As I mentioned earlier, I became a teacher shortly before yoga exploded in popularity in the United States. Riding that wave placed me in a good spot for a successful career, so I feel very lucky.

- *Financial security:* You've probably met a teacher who manages her money well or has money in the bank already. Sometimes people like this succeed as teachers simply because they are not nervous or uptight about finances and have greater access to training, clothing, and resources that enhance their career.
- *Innate physical prowess:* Instagram features endless pictures of naturally bendy yogis — often former gymnasts, acrobats, athletes, or martial artists — who have built huge social media followings because of their physical capability. Whether they were born exceptionally flexible and strong or worked hard to get that way, having a bendy, advanced asana practice can be a source of inspiration to students and increase one's chances of success.
- *Gender:* Although this might sound cynical, being a male yoga teacher in a mostly woman-dominated market has its advantages. While there are millions of successful and popular women yoga teachers, men can sometimes be more popular at the studio simply because they are something of a novelty.
- *Fashion sense:* A distinct and clear personal style or fashion sense can be an advantage, enhancing a teacher's most attractive features and making her stand out in the crowd.
- *Marketing acumen:* While marketing and social networking skills can be cultivated and learned, some people just have a knack for technology and a natural affinity for marketing and promotion. Using social media comes easily to these people. Of course, many successful yogis eschew technology, preferring to base their teaching and their business on face-to-face personal relationships. The fact remains, however, that many yogis who are adept at social media and marketing are building monumental followings that help their classes fill more quickly, land endorsement deals, and garner paid partnerships in exchange for shout-outs. (In fact, some yogis are earning more through social media than through teaching!).
- *Compelling background:* Some yoga teachers have survivor stories, meaning that they survived something tragic or difficult in life that people relate to. Students will often seek help with a similar challenge in their own lives by studying with such a teacher. I don't wish any kind of survivor story on anyone, but for teachers who are

willing to share the wisdom gained from such an experience, it can help draw students.
- *Yoga pedigree:* Some students seek out yoga teachers who have studied directly under legendary teachers like B. K. S. Iyengar, Pattabhi Jois, or their disciples. Because a connection to a very well-known yoga teacher can increase your own visibility, training and apprenticing with such a teacher is not only effective for your education but also potentially helpful for your career later on.

Identifying Areas of Potential Improvement

In reviewing these definitions of skilled, exemplary, and successful teachers, you've probably recognized aspects of yourself and areas where you excel. I hope you also contemplate changes and improvements you'd like to make in your practice, teaching, and career and the goals you want to pursue. The easiest way to start improving is to highlight some of the qualities listed above that you could enhance, and then take action to fill in the gaps.

For example, to become more skilled, would you benefit from training with a different teacher or at a more advanced level? Could you videotape your class so that you can watch yourself and look for ways to refine your teaching?

To work toward becoming exemplary, could you be more honest with your students about the fact that you actually do enjoy a glass of wine on occasion, or could you work on building more community and encouraging conversation with students by inviting them on a group outing after class?

To consider ways you might become more successful, let's do a more detailed self-assessment and look at how to define your core values, which are the basis of your mission statement and the choices and goals you make for yourself and your career.

Discovering Your Core Values

Successful companies orient themselves around a clear set of core values. So can yoga teachers! Core values are the fundamental beliefs or principles that drive your actions. They are what makes you tick and what truly inspires you. To get your set of core values clear, you must be able to explore — with ruthless honesty — what matters most in your life.

Knowing your core values helps define who you are as a person and as a professional. These values consciously and unconsciously drive your decision making in every aspect of your life. If you orient your life around your core values, there is no need to push yourself to be motivated or to spend too long agonizing over decisions: your values will motivate and guide you. In addition, connecting to your core values will help you:

- be more passionate about your teaching
- be more authentic
- build your student base and find colleagues and partners who share your values
- be clear about your future path and make strategic decisions for your career
- stay focused on what matters most in your life and career

Determining what your core values are is fairly easy; living by them, however, takes courage. Among other things, it means being willing to say no to opportunities that don't align with your values. For example, if you don't agree with the values of a studio where you've been offered work, living by your core values will mean turning down the offer — and the potential income.

Sticking to your values also means being able to withstand criticism. Some people will share and endorse your values, and others will find them unattractive. If your values are obviously pushing lots of other people's buttons, you might want to reconsider your reasoning or your self-presentation. However, even if your values are authentic and truly yours (and not those you've passively absorbed from others), and you are striving to live by them, you will likely encounter at least a little disagreement. But I've found that stirring up a bit of controversy isn't a bad thing. One example is a video made by our team at 90 Monkeys in response to the "Shit Girls Say" video that went viral. Our variation on the theme, "Shit Unprofessional Yoga Teachers Say," was definitely controversial, but it has received close to a hundred thousand views and brought a lot of traffic to our site.

If you have the courage, living by your core values will distinguish you as a leader and a teacher. Your bravery will be rewarded by energy and passion in your yoga career.

COMMON CORE VALUES

Here are some examples of our graduates' values:

- Responsibility
- Leadership
- Respect
- Community
- Integrity
- Generosity
- Space
- Creativity
- Grace
- Dignity
- Educating others
- Having fun
- Having an impact
- Uplifting
- Service
- Design sense
- Ingenuity
- Setting standards
- Nurturing
- Support
- Quest
- Excellence
- Mastery

There are a number of ways to come up with your list of core values. Five is a good number to aim for. One way is to talk to the people closest to you. These should be people who know you well and who you trust to be honest with you. Run a few words or phrases by them and get their feedback. For example, you may think of authenticity and generosity as two of your core values. Other people can let you know if your actions are typically in line with those concepts and whether you "walk your talk."

You can also try this exercise in reverse, inferring your values from your actions rather than checking to see if your actions match your stated ideals. Think of two or three choices or decisions you've made recently. Look at the action you ultimately took and think about what values it reveals. For example, if you passed up a promotion that would have entailed moving across the country, you may have been influenced by your spouse's career, your children's education, or the needs of your aging parents. What values does this choice reveal? If, instead, you chose to take the job, what values did that decision reflect?

Another exercise that I found very helpful comes from a seminar with success coaches Jim Bunch and Jack Canfield. Describe the following scenarios to a trusted friend or mentor, and have them jot down key words you use while you tell your stories. Don't overthink what you are saying, and keep each story to about two minutes.

1. Consider a time in your life when everything was going well for you, a time that you look back at and say, "That was the best time of my life!"
2. Consider a time in your life when you were devastated and nothing was going well for you.

Ask your friend to tally how many times you repeat the same words or concepts as you tell the two stories. In the second part of the exercise, some of the words you use will be negative, the opposites of your values. For example, if you repeat a phrase like "I felt like I was alone and had no friends," it probably reflects that one of your core values is community and friendship. The words you've used the most are bound to reflect your core values.

You can also contemplate your values by yourself, writing down your thoughts, or look at the ways other people have approached this question. In his *Autobiography*, Benjamin Franklin listed thirteen virtues he aspired to live by. They're listed on the website ThirteenVirtues.com.

Understanding Why You Teach

The mission statement is a succinct, one- or two-sentence statement about the nature and purpose of your business. Before you try to write yours, I encourage you to think deeply about specifically why you teach yoga. (You may find it interesting to jot down an answer now, and then another after answering the questions below.)

After writing my own mission statement as a yoga teacher, I discovered that on days when I was not inspired to teach, if I simply recalled my highest reason for teaching, I could instantly think of a focus for the class or a theme I wanted to share. I'd get energized and look forward to seeing who'd be in the studio, and I was much more eager to motivate my students to express themselves in their poses.

Why do you teach yoga? Ask yourself the following questions:

- Why does your yoga business exist?
- How does it benefit people?
- If you were not teaching yoga, what would the world miss out on?
- What skills were you born with?
- What are your unique talents?
- What do you feel you were born to do on this planet?
- Why do you personally love to teach yoga?

SOME ANSWERS FROM OUR TRAINEES

- If you were not teaching yoga, what would the world miss out on?
  Kindness
  Community
  Self-love
  Empowerment
  Inspiration
  Self-acceptance
  Reflection
  Healing

Possibility
Self-connection
Fun
Playfulness
A way to tune back in to the body and intuition
An opportunity to be happy about who we are

- What are your unique talents?
  Humor
  Bringing people together
  Building community
  Communicating
  Using themes and metaphors (taking it "off the mat")
  Functional anatomy
  Reminding others that they can shine

- Why do you personally love to teach yoga?
  Seva (service)
  Sharing my gifts
  Getting people to smile
  Yoga changed my life for the better, and I want to share that change
  I want to inspire people
  To make the world a better place
  Yoga gave me peace and I want to give that to others
  I get high from seeing people come back to themselves.

Some people find it hard to compile a list of their talents, especially because some yoga teaching trains us to be humble and to suppress the ego. But not sharing your gifts can be a disservice to the community. And you have to recognize and value your gifts in order to know you have something vital to share. Your relationship with the ego is healthy when you remember the source of your power — the divine. (By contrast, if you think you deserve sole credit for all your skills and talents, then yes, your ego may be a problem.) The more you understand and own the gifts you were born with, the sooner you can start making a difference in this world!

Your Mission Statement

It's time to put your self-reflection and analysis into the form of a concise mission statement. This doesn't have to follow the format of statements found in a traditional business plan. (However, a formal business plan can help you solidify your plan and business, and you will likely need one if you are applying for loans or seeking financial backing for a teaching business.) I think of the mission statement more as a way for us to ground our teaching goals. We know what we are about, and if asked, we can explain our mission clearly to others.

What should a statement look like? It should convey who you are, what you do, what you stand for, and why you do it. It can indicate what kind of people you are serving and what benefits you offer them. Your mission statement should explain why your teaching business exists.

Consider the factors you've identified so far — your teaching strengths and areas of potential improvement, your core values, your reasons for teaching — and write your mission statement with them in mind. This is your chance to envision a world that is transformed through your teaching, a world that benefits from your greatest passions and natural talents. Have fun with it. Give yourself plenty of time to refine your statement, and run it by friends and people who have been influential in your life.

Here is my latest mission statement:

> My mission is to inspire people to experience their interconnection with all of life while reaching their potential in many dimensions: personal, professional, emotional, and spiritual. Through sharing my writing, art, and movement practices, I am here to help others become more conscious, awake, and alive, so that they live on the earth more fully and sustainably — all while courageously having an adventurously good time.

If you are new to teaching, perhaps this is the first time you've tried to put such a statement together. If you are a veteran teacher, you may want to refine a statement you created previously. In any case, it's a good idea to revisit your mission statement every few years, since you are always changing and growing.

Identifying Your Ideal Students and Their Needs

The above exercises are intended to help us understand who we are as teachers, what matters most to us, and what we hope to gain from teaching. But successful teaching — and a successful business — requires two-way interaction. We also need to understand and respect the expectations, abilities, and personal circumstances of our students and teach them in a way that helps them meet their goals. In business terms, we need to identify our market. With so many yoga students out there, we are free to choose which types of students we most enjoy teaching and tailor our business to appeal to them.

In practical terms, what do students want? If you are teaching yoga to a clearly defined group — expectant mothers, back pain sufferers, or cancer survivors — the answer might be obvious. Conversely, among a diverse group, like students at a high-end spa or a local YMCA, we would anticipate a wider range of abilities and expectations.

In general, I have found that students' expectations for a yoga class are often not clearly defined. Beginners want to experience some of the physical, mental, and emotional benefits they have heard about, while more-advanced students often simply want more of the benefits they are already getting from their practice.

As teachers, we need to strike a balance between offering what we think is best for our students (perhaps things they haven't even thought about) and satisfying their expectations.

How do we strike this balance? First and foremost, we listen — and we create an environment that invites conversation, ideally before or after class. Here are some ways to connect with students:

- Take a moment at the start of class to ask not just about a student's familiarity with yoga but also about special concerns.

- Ask students with limitations, injuries, or any other special needs to raise their hands so you can talk to them before class and also check in with them during and afterward.
- Give every brand-new student a questionnaire asking what they hope to gain from yoga and asking them to list any injuries or limitations.

You can't tailor an entire class of twenty students to the particular limitations of one or two, but if you maintain an openness toward students in a mixed-level class, students with special needs will feel comfortable approaching you to discuss them. Make it clear to students that questions are welcome, and encourage them to speak up immediately if anything hurts, so that you can assist the students in their alignment.

In our teacher training workshops, we ask teachers to list what they believe the average yoga student wants out of a yoga class. Here are some of the answers we've received from yoga teachers all over the world:

Kindness
Challenge
To feel good about themselves
To feel better physically and emotionally
Relaxation
Fitness
Flexibility
Connection to community
To feel supported
To move
To feel safe
To improve lives
Time out to relax
Better connection to self
To meet like-minded people
Stress relief
Time for themselves
To restore energy

Yoga Journal's "Yoga in America" study respondents reported the following as the top five reasons for starting and continuing to practice:

1. Flexibility
2. Stress relief/reduction
3. General fitness/conditioning
4. Improvement of overall health
5. Physical fitness

Exploring your mission as a teacher, discovering your core values, and identifying your ideal students and what they need will give you a road map to guide you toward success as a yoga teacher.

Part II

GETTING DOWN TO BUSINESS

CHAPTER THREE

Yoga Business Basics

In the last chapter we addressed the first step to success: defining what you want. The next step is figuring out how to get there. This chapter covers some of the practical aspects of being a yoga teacher: identifying and selecting business channels, building a student base, retaining students, and marketing your skills and talents. If you've been teaching on a fulltime basis for a while, some of this will be familiar and you may wish to either use it as a review or skip ahead.

There are many sources of income for yoga teachers, involving different periods, levels, and types of commitment, and drawing on different business skills. For example, organizing a yoga retreat involves not only planning and teaching classes but also marketing, organizing accommodations and meals, accounting, and administration. Private lessons are based on individual relationships, and workshops are focused on content. Being a yoga professional requires us to juggle many balls, swim in many streams, wear many hats — pick your metaphor.

I can quickly think of eleven business channels:

1. Beginner series/classes
2. Specialty series
3. Group classes
4. Private lessons
5. Workshops
6. Teacher trainings

7. Retreats
8. Conferences and festivals
9. Product sales
10. Partnerships and endorsements
11. Teaching in workplaces and at schools, colleges, and continuing education venues

Let's look more closely at these.

Beginner Series/Classes

What did you think about your first yoga teacher? When I asked yoga teachers this question, most of them reported thinking that their first teacher was the best ever! This teacher was a role model who taught them well and gave them something they value greatly; she got them hooked on the practice. Being a student's first yoga teacher is a privilege — and a responsibility, because a bad first experience with a teacher can turn a student off from yoga forever.

From the perspective of a teacher, it can be very rewarding to help beginners, who are first experiencing the gifts of yoga. From a professional perspective, beginner yoga students are a gift to treasure. If you are not reaching out to the beginner population, you are missing a wonderful opportunity. Students who already do yoga also already have teachers. A bunch of teachers all attempting to teach to the same population of students can work against one another in unnecessary ways. Running a regular beginner series can be a great solution to this problem. Beginner series can be offered monthly, quarterly, or biannually depending on student demand, and each series usually runs for four to eight weeks.

ETIQUETTE GUIDE FOR NEW STUDENTS

On our website, 90Monkeys.com, we offer a comprehensive yoga etiquette guide for new students. At the top of the page, simply subscribe to our online newsletter, and the guide will be emailed to you.

In Boulder, Colorado, where I live, a large percentage of the population practices yoga, and there are also lots of yoga teachers. I've heard many of these teachers complain about the surplus of teachers and the scarcity of students. But even in locations like Boulder, where lots of people do yoga, *there will always be many more who don't (yet)*. Many are curious about yoga and perhaps have a friend who practices. More and more often, doctors are recommending yoga to patients as a way to relieve pain and stress. Athletes have heard it's good for their muscles, and elderly students understand that it can help them maintain their mobility. Recruiting new students from among these populations can spare you from friction with other teachers and enables you to form the special bond between the students and you, as their first teacher. Students like these will stick with you for the long haul: from there they can matriculate into group classes, private lessons, workshops, and all your other offerings.

The practical advantage of teaching a beginner series, or any other kind of series, if you charge in advance, is that you can plan on a specific level of income for an extended period. You can also plan a good part of your schedule ahead of time.

To derive the greatest benefit from this business channel, offer these series regularly throughout the year. In addition, make sure there is a basic or mixed-level class for your graduates to attend when they complete the series so they have a way to continue their practice!

Specialty Series

Whether you're an independent yoga teacher or a studio owner/manager, another way to reach students who may not already be practicing yoga regularly, or to appeal to current students, is to offer series of classes tailored to specific groups or needs. Some examples include yoga for the lower back, yoga for cyclists, prenatal yoga, yoga for men, or yoga for runners.

PLAYING TO YOUR STRENGTHS

To come up with ideas for series that would be fun and effective for you to teach, brainstorm by making a list of your strengths and interests and match that to possible series topics. For example, you might be naturally inclined toward helping people with injuries and thus could offer a yoga series such as "Yoga for the Lower Back" or "Yoga for Shoulders." Or perhaps you are a gifted athlete in a particular sport. If so, then you can help those in your sport get more freedom through yoga by leading a series called, for example, "Yoga for Runners."

Group Classes

Group classes are the most common income source for yoga teachers. Perhaps the most rewarding aspect of teaching group classes is the sense of community that builds when a group practices together consistently over time.

When you teach at a studio, you'll either be paid a flat fee for your class or be paid "by the head," or per student. Some studios will pay a combination of both.

Being paid by the head places more of the incentive for marketing the class on the teacher, making it a collaborative effort between the studio and the teacher. A flat fee puts the marketing onus only on the studio. Having both parties marketing the class is a win-win.

The advantage of being paid a flat fee is that you can depend on a steady income no matter how many students attend your class. The downside is that flat fees are typically not very high. When paid a flat fee, although you may not make as much income, think of it as a way to build a loyal base of students who will funnel into your workshops, series, or retreats. And as always, consistently show up for class, give students a challenging but safe practice, and do not sub out your class too often!

Private Lessons

Private classes pay the highest hourly rate (after teacher trainings). Although they can be more taxing, especially if you travel to students' homes, four to seven private lessons a week can provide a good, reliable chunk of weekly income. You might want to set a goal of working with a certain number of private clients per week. The intimacy of teaching private lessons can be too intense for some yoga teachers, though, so you might also choose not to offer them.

To build this business channel, keep track of your students' progress in a notebook or file so you are always sharing fresh teachings and have clear boundaries around time. And don't be afraid to invite a student to take private lessons with you!

Workshops

Workshops often take place on a weekend or over a few consecutive weeknights. They can target many of the interest groups mentioned above: pregnant women, athletes, kids, cancer survivors, men, golfers. There's an almost endless variety of opportunities for niche teaching in addition to general options.

To build this channel, survey your regular students about what kinds of things they want to learn more about in yoga. Pay attention to how students respond to what you teach in your regular classes: what teachings do they seem to love, or what poses do they need more practice with? These observations could spark some desirable workshop themes. Then when the time comes to offer a workshop, students will be hungry for what you have to share.

Teacher Trainings

If you have a knack for teaching others the "science" behind how you teach what you teach, teacher training might be a natural evolution for you once you've been teaching yoga for a while. Teacher training has two facets: teaching people to become new yoga teachers and working with existing yoga teachers to improve their teaching skills.

Training other teachers is definitely not for everyone; in fact, there are veteran yoga teachers who are wildly popular but who have rarely, if ever, trained other teachers. It's just not their thing. If teacher training is for you, you'll probably know: you'll feel a natural pull to help others in this capacity, and you might be invited to be part of the faculty for a teacher training. Being invited is always a good sign that others believe in your talents and want what you have to offer.

Teacher training as a business channel pays very well, since professional training tuitions command a higher price than group classes or workshops. Tuition can be higher because it represents an investment for trainees and offers a certification toward a career path. And when you've gotten to the point in your career that you have enough knowledge and aptitude to teach other teachers, your expertise is worthy of higher compensation.

There are two teacher training business models. First, you can run and administer your own training independently. In this scenario you handle all revenue and pay yourself accordingly after expenses.

Alternatively, you might be on faculty through a studio or other organization, which is more typical for newer teachers. In this case, you are less involved in the marketing of the training, and there are a couple of ways you can be compensated. The first way is to set an hourly rate for your time. Typically this is twice what you would charge hourly for private lessons. The second compensation option is based on the projected revenue from the training program and the number of students who enroll. For trainings hosted by a third-party studio, the typical arrangement is to split the net profits 60:40 or 70:30 in favor of the teacher. If you teach only part of the training, you can ask to be paid a fee proportional to the part you teach. For example, if you teach 5 hours of a 180-hour training, that represents 2.7 percent (5÷180) of the total hours. Calculate this percentage of the net profit and then split it 70:30 with the studio.

In order to cultivate teacher training as a business channel, listen to your intuition as to whether teacher training is for you. If it is, prepare well, and be very realistic about managing students' expectations. Students invest a lot more in teacher training than other programs, so rather than promising all kinds of perks and outcomes and then underdelivering because the demands of the training were too much for you to handle, promise "low" and then overdeliver.

Retreats

Retreats are a fantastic way to build community, take your students deeper into the practice, and get away to an exotic location. They involve a great deal of work before, during, and after — but, hey, you get to spend time in a beautiful spot and maybe tack on a vacation if you can spare the time! Because of the planning required and the expenses of renting a facility, retreats are not always financially lucrative, but the finances can work out well if you have a large number of students who want to travel with you. When your students have a good time, they are more likely to become long-term clients, so despite the hard work retreats require, they can be a reasonable investment in your community and career.

To excel with retreats, think about hiring an assistant to help you oversee the retreat administration and ensure that your students are well taken care of. Like a teacher training program, a retreat is a high-ticket item for participants, so make sure you manage expectations well.

Conferences and Festivals

Teaching at events such as conferences and festivals will give you good visibility and potentially attract new students. However, to be invited to teach at such an event, you need a fairly well-established reputation and a loyal student base. Again, because of the preparation time, travel, and teaching time involved, the financial reward may not be all that high.

If you're serious about building this business channel, be prompt in all your dealings and emails with festival organizers and stay on top of marketing tasks. Answering emails and providing workshop descriptions in a timely manner go a long way. Yoga teachers who are unresponsive do not get asked back.

Product Sales

The market for yoga products such as instructional materials, props, clothing, bags, and other accessories is huge. You can benefit by creating your own yoga product or selling someone else's product on your website or in person. However, selling products during classes can be a sensitive issue, since students have paid money for your teaching and may not be receptive to sales pitches. Furthermore, creating any pressure for students to buy products may represent an abuse of the teacher-student relationship. Whether you are comfortable selling things in or around yoga classes depends on how you feel about yoga and consumerism. My personal take is that yoga cannot shelter us from the fact that we are consumers, any more than we can stop outside noise from happening when we meditate. Therefore, if you are excited to sell cool products to support your students' practices as part of this business channel, go for it — just do it tastefully and tactfully. Choose products you can be comfortable endorsing, sourced from vendors that offer sustainably manufactured yoga products.

Partnerships and Endorsements

With the many competing brands of yoga-related clothing, props, and accessories now available, many companies rely on yoga teachers to promote their products, much like big apparel and equipment brands sponsor athletes. You may already be doing it for free if you've worn an outfit or sported a prop and had one of your students or colleagues approach you and ask, "Where did you get that?" Modeling products is effective marketing.

Many of these sellers will approach yoga teachers who are well regarded in their communities about becoming an "ambassador." Most will ask a teacher to wear or display their merchandise in exchange for free products and mentioning their name in a blog or a social networking post here and there. Such relationships are typically not exclusive: you can still wear and use other brands. If you have a large enough number of social media followers and influence, however, you can sometimes negotiate an exclusive promotional arrangement with a brand, by which you agree to use only their products in your teaching and public appearances in exchange for a fee.

If you're hoping to develop this channel, the key is to be patient. You'll also want to establish yourself as a thought leader in the field, which means writing articles and blogs and building a robust social media following on platforms like Facebook, Instagram, and Twitter.

Teaching in Workplaces and at Schools

Teaching workplace yoga, or "corporate yoga," as it is sometimes called, can be extremely fulfilling. You can make a huge difference in employees' comfort, health, and productivity. For employees who sit hunched over their computers for hours with endless deadlines to meet, you are a breath of fresh air! You can teach a variety of poses to counter the effects of sitting, "computer neck," low back pain, and hunched shoulders that afflict millions of workers, as well as teaching them breathing, meditation, and other mindfulness techniques to help boost their productivity and consciousness.

Corporate yoga instruction can be set up in two ways. First, it can be arranged through a wellness agent in your area who acts as a sort of broker, connecting companies with wellness experts and fitness trainers. If you can find such a broker or business, you can drop off your résumé or offer them complimentary classes so that they can see how you teach. If you're a fit, they can start placing you with companies looking to bring yoga into their facilities.

When I first started teaching, I was lucky enough to have such an agent come to a class at the studio where I taught. After taking my class, she brought me on board immediately, and from there I went on to teach executives at Atlantic Records, Bear Stearns, and Pfizer. I am still in touch with some of the students I taught, and some even went on to become yoga teachers!

The second way to arrange corporate yoga classes is to set up the program yourself directly with the company. For me, this happened organically when students attending my group classes approached me about teaching in their workplace. One of the coolest programs I organized was teaching the cast and crew of the Broadway show *Beauty and the Beast*. "The Beast" was a regular in my group classes and asked me to come to the theater to teach!

Many companies are looking for relatively low-cost ways to offer employee benefits and decrease health-care costs, and yoga classes are appealing on both counts. The best way to approach a company is through its human resources department, whose staff can get the word out to employees.

When you are arranging a corporate program, you'll want to ask who is paying: will the employees be covering the classes, or is the company willing to offer the classes to employees as a perk? Or perhaps the company is willing to pay for half of the class fee while the employee covers the rest.

The most straightforward option is for the company to cover the entire cost and compensate you directly. In this case, you should charge what you would for teaching a private class in a client's home, plus 10 to 20 percent to cover multiple students. However, not all businesses can afford to offer their employees free yoga classes. Either way, it's best if the human resources department handles your payment. If the employees pay part of the class fee, the company can determine what to charge, based on your flat fee, and collect the fee from them.

There are other ways to handle pricing and compensation, such as being paid by the head, but the above methods require the least amount of administrative work on your part.

Teaching yoga in schools or other educational venues requires networking. Again, students in your regular group classes might approach you about opportunities to lead yoga classes in their club, school, or gym. If you are a parent, you might talk with the teachers at your children's school about offering yoga. You can follow the same approach to pricing and compensation that we recommend above for corporate yoga, keeping in mind that budgets may not be as high as in corporate settings.

Doing the Numbers

When you're deciding how and how much you want to teach, it's helpful to sit down and think hard about your personal and financial situation. First, look at how much money you *need* to live and pay your expenses. Then consider how much income you *want* in order to be, do, and have everything you value in life. This, of course, brings up the question of whether a yoga teacher's income can ever really cover all that we want to be, do, and have. My answer is that yoga may never fulfill our wildest financial dreams, but it can provide a decent annual income with the freedom to create your own schedule and work on your own terms. And if it doesn't meet your financial needs or desires completely, you may have to supplement it with a day job and/or pursue other ways of earning part of your living. The key is to maximize what you can earn, and that takes foresight and planning.

As a professional, you want to look at the different channels available to you, assess which ones are your strongest and weakest sources of income, and then determine whether you'd like to add a new channel or improve a channel that could be more lucrative.

If you are interested in adding a new business channel, a first step is to visualize yourself succeeding at it. You can add it as a symbol on your altar or *puja* where you meditate, even if it is just a phrase on a sticky note like "I am leading a beautiful retreat in Mexico." Next, take action toward augmenting the channels that interest you most. For example, take a course on how to offer a retreat, go on a retreat yourself, or attend a variety of workshop events to see what it would be like. Ask for help from other teachers who have done it before.

When refining business channels you already have in place, examine how well you are managing all aspects of that source of income. Are your classes consistently well attended? If not, consider what you might change. Are they offered at appealing times? Do people know about the classes? Are they enthusiastically promoted, and is that promotion targeted in savvy ways? Think about the quality of your teaching. If we're honest, most of us know if we routinely fall short in some way.

Once you have determined which business channels you want to focus on, start making specific plans, such as how many times a year you want to offer programs like specialty series, retreats, and workshops. Balance these with your regular weekly commitments, like group classes and private lessons.

Last, map out these offerings on your yearly calendar and then create a marketing plan (see page 90) to ensure that each event and ongoing offering is a success. Whether you plan to implement these offerings immediately or are planning for the future, you can map out the entire year and estimate an annual income that accommodates your needs and wants.

Creating a Balanced Teaching Schedule

If you are a new teacher, it's best to refine your teaching by focusing on your group classes. You might also start working to build your private clientele and plan ahead for offering a beginner series in your area.

A nicely balanced schedule at this point might look something like this:

Ongoing Offerings

- *Private lessons:* Four lessons per week
- *Group classes:* Eight to fifteen classes per week

Beginner Series

- Monthly or every other month

As you advance, you become ready to start leading workshops, retreats, or specialty series. I knew I was ready to handle these extra offerings when two things started to happen:

1. My students asked me to lead more in-depth workshops and started requesting that I take them on retreat to an exotic locale.
2. Studio owners invited me to teach a workshop, and I was invited to colead a teacher training.

As I mentioned earlier, when people begin to invite you to do things, it's probably a sign that you're ready and the demand is there. Although it is possible to start offering workshops or retreats before being asked, I can guarantee that offerings will be more successful, and you will feel more confident and well received, if someone else has invited you first. From a marketing perspective, if someone invites you, they will actively support your efforts. If you invite yourself, they may have less enthusiasm because it was your idea, not theirs.

REMEMBER YOUR OWN ONGOING EDUCATION

As you plan your teaching offerings, it's important to allow time and resources for your own ongoing education. I like to include some form of continuing education for myself at least once a quarter, whether that is an in-person event or some kind of online learning. The kind of program you choose is up to you; it needs to fit your budget and your personal and teaching obligations. Obviously online learning is less expensive and more convenient than traveling somewhere to take a class. However, nothing can replace the experience of being in the same room with other students and a teacher who can observe you in person. Either way, I recommend budgeting 5 to 10 percent of your income for continuing education! Prioritize this kind of savings commitment for education, even when it seems impossible: it is vital for keeping you fresh and inspired and ultimately boosting your business.

If you are a seasoned teacher who is ready to teach or already teaching workshops, retreats, and specialty series, continually add events to your schedule. Also, you might teach fewer ongoing group classes and devote more time to other, more financially rewarding offerings. You might set up a target schedule like the following:

Specialty Series/Classes and Retreats

Beginner series: Four to six per year (seasonal)
Workshops: Four per year (seasonal)
Full retreat: One weeklong winter getaway to an exotic locale
Long-weekend retreats: One or two seasonal mini-getaways per year
Specialty series: Two to four per year
Fund-raiser benefit classes: One to three per year

Ongoing Offerings

- *Private lessons:* Four to six lessons per week
- *Group classes:* Six to ten classes per week

GIFT CERTIFICATES

One way to promote offerings such as private lessons, beginner series, and specialty series is to offer holiday or special-occasion gift certificates. The December holidays are a great opportunity!

Five Steps to Building a Solid Student Base

As part of yoga business basics, I advise my clients to think about how to develop a strong student base. I have boiled it down to a five-step process through which teachers reach students and inspire them to come to class, stay with the practice, and become loyal to the practice — and to you, as their teacher.

The five steps may not sound "yoga-like." That's because we borrowed them from corporate/business terminology. We use them because it's helpful to have language to describe this process, but we do not mean to cheapen the experience or to commodify students! The results of applying this five-step process go back to our highest vision: more people doing yoga to help build a more conscious world.

1. Identify and Reach

The first step in the process is to identify the types of students you want to teach. You might think of them according to occupation: office workers, school teachers, nurses, military personnel, or stay-at-home parents. Or you might think about categories of needs: new moms, athletes, children, people with chronic pain, people in recovery, or people with depression or anxiety. You can probably identify many more categories.

To reach a group of potential students, you must consider what that group most wants. Can you provide it? This is the *value proposition*.

For example, if you are reaching out to parents with new babies, what would be the value of yoga to a new mother or father? Possibilities include:

Time for themselves

Rehabilitating the body after pregnancy
Better sleep
Cultivating patience
Cultivating gentleness
Accepting imperfection
Encouraging body acceptance
Companionship with other new parents
Confidence to step into a new life
Community

Once you've identified your target group, think about how you could reach out to them. For new parents, possible points of contact include:

Pediatric offices
Midwives/doulas
Baby stores
Breastfeeding groups
Parent support groups
Mom-and-baby groups
Kindergartens
Day care centers
Playgroups and other children's activities
Schools
Social networking groups
Coffee shops

Now, let's look at how to serve a much different population: athletes. You might reason that they want:

Better performance in a sport
Cross training
Balance improvement
Injury prevention and recovery
Increased body awareness
Flexibility
Improved focus
Enhanced recovery from training
Pain relief

Places where you could reach this group include:

- Workplaces
- Physical therapy offices
- Running groups
- Cycling groups
- Facebook groups
- Orthopedic offices
- Health clubs
- Sporting events (races, games, competitions)
- Sporting goods retailers

For these two groups, both the value propositions and the possible points of contact are dramatically different (even though some individuals might fit in both categories!). This difference illustrates how much skill and awareness is involved in reaching new clients.

When you've identified the value proposition that aligns most closely with your students' needs, your programming becomes much more effective. Now you can convey that value proposition clearly in your promotional materials, in social media posts, and in person when you announce your events and programs. You'll be able to qualify the benefits of your offering in such a way that students will want to say yes to signing up. When you're teaching, you can target your yoga classes so that they're specifically geared toward your students' needs and desires.

2. Acquire

Acquiring a student refers to the moment when someone signs up for one of your classes. The exact acquisition process will depend on where you are teaching. It may require the student to register at the facility, sign up for specific classes, complete waivers or questionnaires and health forms, and arrange payment. If you are an independent teacher working at a studio, the studio may handle most of this process.

The acquisition period often forms the first (and most lasting) impression for students; it's imperative to make sure they are welcomed and given a proper orientation to the facility and the class. For example, it is customary to show new students where they can change and leave their belongings, where the bathrooms are, and how to get props and a towel if they need them. This can be an overwhelming time for a new student and frequently for the teacher as well. The student may be completely unfamiliar with yoga and feel intimidated in a new environment. The teacher may be inundated with questions from new students while trying to prepare for class. This is a key moment to model remaining poised, calm, inviting, and reassuring.

During the Acquire phase (and actually during all phases), it is imperative to respond to prospective students in a timely manner. When you get back to students quickly, it leaves a very good impression and you will be more likely to see positive results in registrations and sales. It seems the busier those in customer care become, the rarer it is to find businesses whose response time is swift. Being responsive and timely will help you stand out in the crowd.

3. Teach

Do your absolute best to engage new students through being prepared and present in your teaching. Draw on all the qualities discussed in chapter 2 that make you a skilled and exemplary teacher.

Teach in a creative, innovative, and dynamic way that makes students want to return. You want your students to get great results. Constantly hone your craft by staying current in your own yoga studies and education.

4. Retain

You know you have good overall retention when your class has a core of regular students. The reason they keep coming every week is that your class has become an integral part of their lives and schedules. You want that core group to grow.

What fosters retention? Outstanding teaching is most important, but other small things can go a long way. These include addressing students by name, giving hands-on adjustments, building relationships outside class, and not subbing out your class too often.

5. Build Loyalty

Loyalty is related to retention, but it's more personal: it means the student would choose your class or studio, even over other teachers' offerings at more convenient times or locations, because they feel they have received so much from you. A connection with a loyal student may be lifelong; it's a relationship almost like what you have with family. It comes from deep bonding experiences through yoga. I have shared some heartfelt moments and adventures with students on retreat that connect us for life.

Here are some ways to build loyalty:

- Text students if you haven't seen them for a while, tell them you've missed them, and ask if they are okay.
- Invite students to community events like movie nights, potlucks, and holiday celebrations.
- Remember to ask clients about their lives rather than talking about your own.
- Remember and celebrate birthdays.
- Recognize students' achievements inside and outside the classroom.

Understanding these five steps to building a student base should give you a good overview of a client's journey from finding you to enjoying your teaching to becoming a long-term, devoted student. To encourage students to be a part of your yoga community for years to come, the key is to be aware of where your students are in this cycle and to continually follow the approaches suggested above.

CHAPTER FOUR

Building Your Business

The practical business issues discussed in the next two chapters may not be new to you if you're already teaching. But if you're reading this book, I assume you want to build your business. Whether you're new to teaching or a veteran, it's beneficial to understand these fundamentals and review them regularly.

Write a Business Plan

First of all, don't panic! The term *business plan* sounds formal, complex, and intricate, but it doesn't have to be. Simply put, a business plan identifies a demand in the marketplace and explains how you plan to fulfill it. My favorite guide is *The One Page Business Plan*, by Jim Horan. It's an easy-to-use workbook that helps solidify your plan and business.

As noted in chapter 2, you may not *need* a formal business plan unless you are applying for loans or seeking financial backing for a teaching business. But your business will feel more solid and professional when you take the time to write up even a simple plan.

Beyond putting a plan on paper, it is also useful to occasionally revisit your mission statement and core values. This helps keep you focused.

HIRE MONEY PROFESSIONALS

You can't hide your head in the sand — or up in a cloud — when it comes to taxes and bills. Unless you are gifted at accounting and bookkeeping, hand these tasks over to professionals. The right accountant and bookkeeper will help you make sense of all money matters including your taxes, knowing what you can write off as business expenses, and getting your bills paid on time.

Neglecting financial matters hurts your teaching in the long run. It can distract you with worry and, at worst, cost you time and money when you have to deal with mistakes and missteps. The best way to find a financial professional you can trust is by word of mouth: ask those closest to you for recommendations.

Build a Yoga Résumé

Keep an up-to-date résumé that describes your training, teaching experience, and special skills and attributes. Have it ready to send out (or to print out and deliver in person) whenever an attractive teaching opportunity arises. The networking site LinkedIn (which you may want to consider signing up for if you haven't already) has its own online résumé form that prompts you to key in relevant items.

List your educational history, including degrees and continuing education certifications. Give details of your yoga training credentials, such as what teacher trainings you graduated from and your main teachers. If you have a Registered Yoga Teacher credential from Yoga Alliance, state the level (RYT 200, RYT 500, E-RYT 200, or E-RYT 500).

For your teaching experience, outline how long you've been a self-employed yoga teacher and describe the types of teaching you've done: for example, "Self-employed yoga teacher, 1997 to present, teaching private lessons, group classes, workshops, retreats, specialty series, and teacher trainings." Specify where you have taught and for how long. It can be useful to tailor your résumé to reflect the values and goals of the specific studio you're applying to. And be sure to include any other skills you possess that are relevant to yoga, such as physical therapy, nursing, psychotherapy, or massage.

Get the Best Teaching Opportunities

I interviewed studio owners and gym managers about how they find their teachers. After doing so, I came up with a list of what teachers can do if they want to pick up classes at a particular studio.

The key is to be present and visible at your desired location. When you are out of sight, it's easy for you to be out of mind. Studio owners and managers have a lot going on and can easily forget about you, even though they might love to have you on the team. Here are some ways to increase your visibility and presence.

- Get on the substitute list by auditioning, if applicable, or dropping off a résumé.
- Guest teach and substitute teach as often as you can at the places where you want to work.
- Attend classes and events where you want to teach.
- Be friendly, helpful, and upbeat. Offer to put away props, fold blankets, or blow out candles at the end of class.
- Make time before and after class to have conversations and build relationships with the staff.
- When you teach as a guest or substitute, ask students at the end of class to recommend you if they enjoyed the class. Say something like, "If you enjoyed class today, please let the management know." This is not too much to ask, and it has worked for me every time. Tell your students how to submit the feedback if it is unclear. For example, you might suggest that they fill out a comment card or mention your teaching to a manager.
- Dress professionally on your way to and from the yoga studio. I suggest wearing regular clothes rather than yoga clothes; after all, you don't often see doctors walking around town in scrubs or white coats! Wear something in which you feel confident, professional, and successful. Active wear, while comfortable, does not exude professionalism.
- When you truly connect with a teaching venue, say so. Let the managers and staff know that you understand and agree with their

values, vibe, and community. Let them know that you are a good fit for their establishment.

When starting out at a studio, you may have to agree to whatever teaching slots the management is willing to give you, but if you are patient and committed to both teaching and marketing, your classes will eventually fill and do well. My rule of thumb is to give it at least four to six months, even if your classes are small. The individualized attention you can provide in smaller classes turns into great word-of-mouth referrals. More important, over time the studio will recognize your efforts and offer you more favorable time slots, and you will feel more confident in asking for them.

When you want to be considered for a better slot at an existing location, here are some steps to take:

- Set a goal for filling the classes you do have, and take action (using the ideas in this book) to increase your student base. It can be frustrating when a time slot is less than ideal, but if you can do the best you can with the slot you currently have, you're more likely to get a better slot sooner.
- Continue to present yourself professionally. Make sure what you wear to, from, and in the studio is clean and looks fresh. This may be hard to do if you're racing around town teaching multiple classes, but a harried, disheveled teacher is hard to rally behind.
- Build relationships with the owners and staff by sharing incidents or issues at the studio they might want to know about. Do so in a supportive way. For example, you might overhear students talking in the changing room about how the studio always smells like sweat right after the 6:00 PM class when they walk in for your restorative class. This is feedback the studio needs to hear, and perhaps it's something that has been bugging you as much as it bugs the students. Relate the feedback in a way that conveys the facts without any emotions you might have attached. Suggest a solution, if you have one, and offer to help implement it.
- Be dependable, willing to work with the studio's vision, open to feedback, and appreciative when you receive feedback.
- Be proactive. Figure out what the studio needs from you and provide it to the best of your ability.

- Follow studio protocols, and if you're going to miss a class, find a good sub ahead of time.
- Be on time, be consistent, and don't miss too many classes.
- Clearly express the ideal class times you'd like to be considered for when they open up, but avoid coming across as impatient or entitled. Instead of saying something like, "I really thought I'd have better slots on the schedule by now," or, "I've been teaching here for two years — don't you think it's time for me to get a 6:00 PM class?," as you build relationships and become closer to the owners, share your vision of how many classes a week you see yourself teaching and what you want to offer your students. Share your vision, values, and mission statement.
- Work with everyone as a team to help the studio succeed, including your fellow teachers. Help build community and synergy.

RURAL BUSINESS BUILDING

Building a yoga community in rural areas can be challenging but, hey, so is yoga! Go ahead and set the ambitious goal of getting everyone in the area into yoga. You might begin by creating a Facebook yoga group for the area to get people talking about yoga, you, and yoga events in your area. Because many people may be new to yoga, be sure to offer accessible beginner classes. As you meet people, remember to add them to your email list and stay in touch.

Try to think of creative, community-specific ways to make your yoga classes must-attend events. Promote them as socializing opportunities for people who may live far apart. Honor someone or something significant in the area and allow students to network about what they do in the community.

Offering tea and light snacks after class is a thoughtful touch that recognizes some people may have traveled a long distance to get to class. Gestures like this count and help you stand out from other teachers. Make your class worth the drive. Respect your students' time by preparing thoroughly to offer classes that give them value.

Should You Quit Your Day Job?

No one ever said being a yoga teacher would make you rich — and if someone does say that, you should probably run away as fast as you can — but it is realistic to believe that yoga can provide a modest living for a single person or a supplementary income for a family. Considering that you may never have to work nine to five, sit in a cubicle, or answer to a boss, you can get by and be pretty happy in the process if you're able to support yourself through teaching.

The yoga lifestyle can be costly, though. Yogis often must travel and pay for continuing education. They tend to be conscious consumers who spend more to support local businesses and humanely and sustainably manufactured products. Like anyone else, they want to support and educate their children well. Many donate generously to good causes. Can a career as a yoga teacher really support this kind of lifestyle?

The answer is that it depends. Some yoga teachers living in urban areas can do quite well with a loyal student base at a popular studio and an affluent clientele who can afford private lessons. Others in different locations struggle to get by.

Once you know how much you need to meet all these expenses, create an annual teaching calendar (as described in chapter 3) and do some projections to estimate your annual income from teaching yoga. If your projected income falls short of your expenses, it's not yet time to quit your day job.

If your current job keeps you from putting 100 percent of your energy into your yoga career, it can be hard to know whether you could safely switch to teaching yoga full time. In this situation it is best to continue to refine your yoga teaching and business skills as a second career until you can be confident that you would do well as a full-time yoga teacher. The fantasy of roaming the world as a yogi, teaching, studying, and answering to no one, is not realistic. A good yogi is also grounded and practical.

Bottom line? Don't quit your day job if it would mean putting yourself or your family on shaky ground.

Sustainable Teaching

Ideally, teaching yoga should be a career that enables you to do what you love while at the same time being able to *live*. An ideal teaching schedule allows ample time for your practice, personal development, leisure pursuits, and time with family and friends. It lets you teach at the times of day when you are most energized, and in locations that enable you to reach the student demographic you serve best and most enjoy teaching.

Often, however, the yoga teacher is more frazzled and unbalanced than her students! Trying to maintain an unsustainable teaching schedule can lead to burnout, resentment, lack of time for practice or professional enrichment, and financial difficulties. For new teachers, the temptation to say yes to every chance to teach can be counterproductive. And agreeing to teach for very little will undermine the market value for all yoga teachers — so be careful not to spread yourself too thin for little compensation.

Every opportunity involves trade-offs. Here are some factors to consider when deciding whether to pursue a teaching opportunity at a studio — or continue with your existing classes there.

- *Exposure and fulfillment:* Consider the studio. Do you like teaching there? Does it have a good vibe, or is there unresolvable tension? Are you nourished and fulfilled by teaching this particular group of students? Is the class size stable or growing? Are you getting good exposure to new students or teaching students who may want to take your workshops and attend your retreats in the future? If so, these factors may offset other potential disadvantages of the class location or schedule.
- *Location:* Traveling to inconvenient locations can be hellish not only for you but also for your students. If that's the case, everyone will be harried as they enter class. Travel delays that cause late arrivals make everyone stressed and apologetic. Classes that are logistically challenging because of travel time or a shortage of parking won't be as well attended. Some of these disadvantages may be offset if the

studio is in a location where you (and your students) can also run errands, get groceries, eat a nice meal, and work out at your favorite gym.
- *Payment models:* As mentioned earlier, studios typically pay either by the class or by the number of students. When you are first starting out and have not yet developed a student base, getting paid by the class is much more secure. However, when you are paid by the number of students, you have greater earning potential and have more incentive to promote your own classes.
- *Student base:* The overall number of students where you're considering teaching can affect your income. A studio with a large student base will be more difficult and competitive to break into. Although you may immediately start off with larger classes, more established studios have a huge number of teachers on their roster. At a newer studio or one with a small student base, it will take longer for you to build your own following, but it might be easier to get desirable teaching slots. So consider whether you can afford to earn less initially by teaching at a studio with a smaller base.

Optimal Scheduling

Long experience, good and bad, has led me to these general guidelines for establishing a productive, sustainable teaching schedule. They involve assessing both the needs of your clientele and your personal situation.

- Traditionally, students tend to prefer attending yoga class every other day with the same instructor for consistency. Be sure you can teach a class at least twice a week at any given studio or gym. Offer classes on alternate days (e.g., Monday and Wednesday or Tuesday and Thursday), in the same style, at the same level, and at the same time at each location. Classes held on consecutive days are not as popular.
- To reach a more diverse crowd, teach various levels of classes, including beginner classes, and teach both daytime and evening classes.
- Tailor your class schedule and offerings to the local community. You can do demographic research at city hall, look up census information

online, or, more simply, observe the places where people are practicing wellness and fitness activities. Do you see mostly women? Men? Athletes? Elderly people? Are there mothers with children in daycare or nursery school? Do you see professionals on a break from the office? When do you see the most people at the gym or wellness center? This information will help you decide which times of day are most convenient for students to attend yoga class, and what types of classes to offer.

- For efficiency, minimize travel between different studios.
- If possible, commit to the time slots when you can be most present and focused. If you're not a morning person, don't say yes to the 6 AM Sunrise Flow! And if you start to fade by 7 PM, say no to the Evening Simmer Down.
- Space your classes so that you have time during the day to eat, rest, practice, do errands, and schedule appointments.
- Schedule private lessons and meetings just before or right after your classes, while you are already out and about.
- Balance your teaching against other important personal commitments, such as date night, family time, yoga class with your favorite teacher, and weekend getaways.
- Miss class only when absolutely necessary. Consistency and presence are critical to the success of your classes. If you're continually having to find substitutes, you don't have the right schedule.
- Keep track of your energy levels. If you can't give your all in every class you teach, consider cutting back or rearranging your schedule.

Some other outside factors influence scheduling preferences. In an area flooded with young professionals and parents with young children, the best-attended classes are often in the late morning, after kids have been dropped off at day care or at school. Parents who need to pick up kids after school are unlikely to attend a 5 PM class. In a downtown area, you'll want to schedule classes around business hours: in the early morning, during lunch breaks, and after 6 PM.

Does class size matter? Of course a smaller class allows more individual attention, and the class can be more easily tailored to the students who are present. On the other hand, a full class is more energizing. We asked our graduates how they taught when the room was full versus sparsely attended in proportion to the size of the room. They said a full class flowed better and that the energy in the room made them more inspired, confident, and engaged. For me, the enthusiasm and increased energy of a full class draws the teachings out of me, and I even come up with new ways of explaining things, resulting in more student engagement. In addition, I have always felt students have a stronger sense of community when they see a full room. Although you might prefer a smaller class with lots of space on the floor, consider how it makes the students feel as well.

A Sustainable Teaching Schedule: A Case Study

During the first "90 Minutes to Change the World" course I ran, one of the teachers asked for my help with her schedule, so I posted her schedule online for everyone to weigh in on. I called it a "fruit-salad schedule" because it was such a random mixture of offerings. It looked like this:

	TUESDAY	THURSDAY
6:00 PM	Level 1/2	Hatha 1
7:15 PM	Power Yoga 1/2	Hatha 2

She taught at a studio Tuesdays and Thursdays. At 6:00 PM she had a Level 1/2, followed by a Power Yoga 1/2. Then on Thursdays she taught Hatha 1, followed by Hatha 2. This schedule made it impossible for a student to attend the same kind of class at the same time every other day. In addition, the names of the classes were confusing: how is Level 1/2 different from Power Yoga 1/2?

Here is the schedule I proposed instead:

	TUESDAY	WEDNESDAY	THURSDAY
6:00 PM	Level 1/2	Power Yoga 1/2	Level 1/2
7:15 PM	Power Yoga 1	Level 2	Power Yoga 1

Scheduling a Level 1/2 class at 6:00 PM and a Power Yoga class at 7:15 PM on Tuesdays and Thursdays would allow students to attend the same-level class regularly. The additional offerings on Wednesday could be paired with Monday or Friday classes. This schedule is much more eye-catching and consistent.

Obviously, if you are an independent teacher, you are not always going to be able to convince the studios or gyms you work for to change their schedules to accommodate you. However, most studio managers want to know about your scheduling vision and may be willing to work with you as time slots open up and change. If you never share your vision, they won't know what you want!

In general, if you are doing very well in a slot, you have the leverage to ask for a schedule change. The irony, of course, is that you might not be doing well in a slot *because* you have a difficult time slot or fruit-salad schedule!

Every relationship with a studio owner or gym manager is going to be different. Be sensitive and tactful, understanding that they are juggling the needs of many teachers, the needs of their business, and their own personal needs.

Should You Open Your Own Studio?

When you've been running around town from class to class for a while, it's natural to fantasize about opening your own studio and having students come to you. Some people long to establish a place where their yoga community can come together. Whatever your motive, if you find yourself considering running your own studio, be sure to consider the pros and cons:

PROS	CONS
Control of your teaching environment	Burdens of supervising other staff, promoting your business, and managing a physical facility
Possible long-term returns on investment if you create a stable, profitable, reputable, and saleable business	Financial risks of fixed studio expenses and uncertain revenue
Chance to create a yoga community	Legal complexities: employment laws, legal liability
Possibility of creating a self-sustaining business that will allow you to take time off occasionally without losing income	Doing your own marketing and promotion (rather than leaving it to the gym or studio manager)
Independence	More responsibility and stress

The decision to open a studio should be made with realistic and careful deliberation. You must determine whether the area can support a yoga studio (or yet *another* yoga studio!) and whether there are suitable spaces available in your area at a reasonable price. Ultimately the decision needs to come from your heart, and you must trust your intuition and inner guidance on what is right for you.

Once you've figured out what, where, and when you want to teach, the next step is getting the word out about your teaching. Most teachers don't enjoy self-promotion, but it is essential if you're going to make a living teaching yoga. In the next chapter we'll look at how to market what you — and yoga — have to offer, and hopefully learn to love doing it in the process!

CHAPTER FIVE

Marketing Your Business

To serve its clients and grow, every business needs to get the word out about what it offers. But the more I talk to yoga teachers, the more I realize how much marketing is a sticky subject. This stickiness has its roots in two places. The first is the issue of how different people relate to yoga and the material world, as we discussed in chapter 1. The second is the notion that yoga students don't want to think about money: many see yoga as an opportunity to rise above the material and mundane.

Yoga teachers tend to internalize the idea that it's wrong to combine yoga and business. They frequently ask me things like, "Amy, if I put myself on Instagram practicing yoga poses, or create a brand and a website, doesn't that go against yoga's values?"

Yet if your goal is to be a professional yoga teacher and educator (rather than viewing yoga solely as a spiritual and personal quest) then it would behoove you to treat your teaching as you would any other professional endeavor that is financially compensated!

We know yoga improves health and wellness, can help reduce stress, and connects people to spirit. In practical terms, the results decrease health-care costs and even save lives. But if yoga teachers don't inform people about these benefits, how can people discover them? We have something powerful to share, and share we must! It's possible to get that message out with subtlety and elegance.

Spreading the Word about Your Services

Define Your Gifts and Goals

How do you teach most effectively? One on one? In small groups? To a room full of students? Do you work best with children, women, men, or people with special needs? Define your ideal students and craft your promotional materials and strategies to reach out to that kind of student.

Craft Your Unique Message

Once you are clear on your assets and goals, find a way to craft your message that is authentic and totally you — and make it classy. You can't go wrong if your message shares who you are and what you have to offer with sincerity. Your mission statement can be your guide. Given the ethics of yoga, crass marketing that artificially glamorizes or oversells you is not going to cut it. Instead of focusing on yourself, focus on the benefits that students will gain from working with you. Get feedback on your promotional material from close friends and students who know you well before making it public.

Confidently Send Out Your Offering

Be confident and enthusiastic in letting others know what you have to offer, knowing that you are providing a valuable service. Publicize your offerings on a website; on social media platforms; through postcards, flyers, and business cards; and by email. Some people will like them, and some will not. You never know — your message might help change someone's life!

The Marketing Funnel

In business, a "marketing funnel" or "purchase funnel" is often used as a model of the theoretical journey of a customer toward the purchase of a product or service.

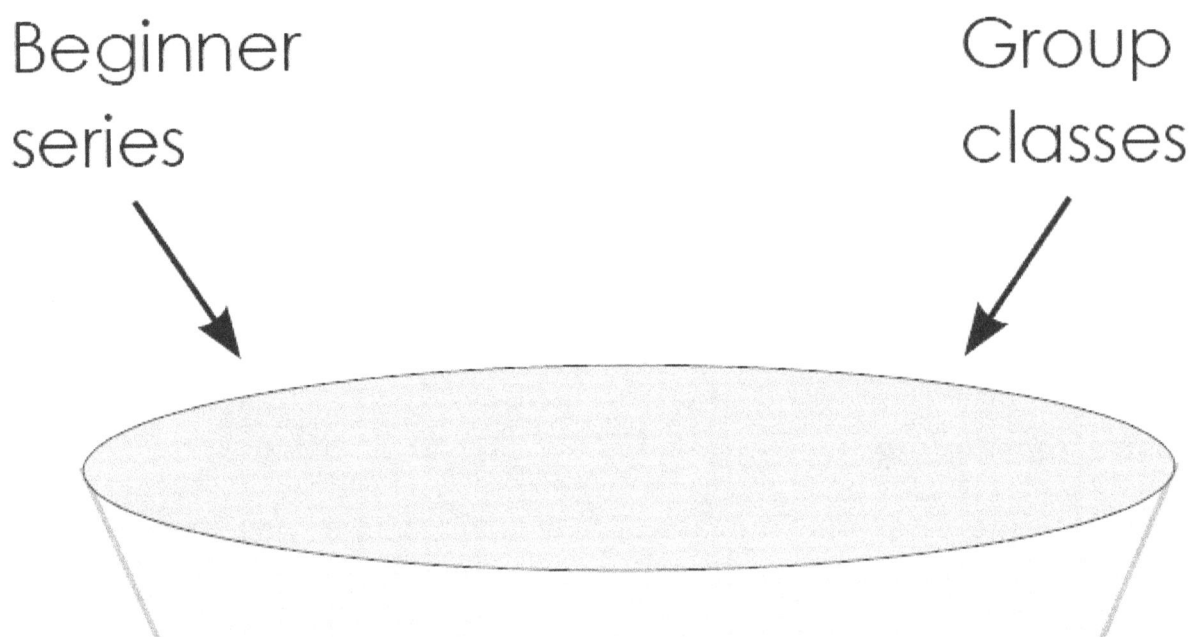

In yoga teaching, the top of the marketing funnel is the entry point to learning yoga. This could be as simple as a flyer for a yoga beginner series pinned on the bulletin board at a coffee shop, or your business cards listing private lessons that people pick up at their chiropractor's office. It could be a popular Facebook post about yoga put up by a yoga studio at which you work. Any of these might lead a beginning student to explore yoga.

As students fall in love with the practice of yoga, they become regulars at classes and begin to seek ways of advancing their practice. These offerings include special workshops, private lessons, specialty series, retreats, and, perhaps, teacher training.

The top of the marketing funnel needs constant attention to ensure a steady flow of new students. Think of it as a stream feeding a lake. If the stream dries up, the lake becomes stagnant. In yoga, this means that teachers are likely to be teaching the same yoga students as their peers are and face a dwindling student base. As existing students move, get sick, pass on, or occasionally lose interest in yoga, it's important to attract a steady stream of new faces.

Creating Your Brand

Brand is a tough word for yoga teachers (and their critics) to swallow. It sounds unspiritual and very corporate. However, if you think more deeply about it, knowing your brand is actually quite in line with yoga principles such as self-inquiry, self-knowledge, and authenticity.

One of the first exercises I give to students who take my training programs is to write down all the things they love about themselves, their talents, their gifts, and their positive assets. Yogis must be able to articulate who they are and their talents. This is not an exercise in narcissism: it is an exercise in knowing your assets so that you can more confidently and freely share your talents with the world. As my teacher Dr. Douglas Brooks once said, "It is a disservice to humanity and your community not to know and share your gifts." To know your assets (as well as your liabilities) is to know your brand.

You don't have to be — and can't be — everyone's yoga teacher. Match your gifts and passions with the student population with whom you want to serve. In other words, be yourself, and you will start to attract the kinds of students you most want to teach.

Knowing your brand, offering teaching that is consistent with your brand, and marketing as your brand actually reduces competition among yoga teachers. Many teachers simply copy what other "successful" teachers are doing, which results in overlap with those other teachers' offerings, instead of doing the self-assessment to gain crystal clarity about their own value propositions. If you are struggling to fill your classes, ask yourself whether you are clear about your brand identity and whether your promotional efforts reflect that identity.

The last time I did a branding inquiry for myself, I asked my students, family, peers, and friends to share words that came to mind when they thought of me. I got responses like *radiant, vivacious, generous with time, knowledgeable, organized*, and *real*.

I then thought about how those words could influence every aspect of my communication with the world, including my font and color choices, photography style, Facebook timeline, Instagram images, the writing style on my website, my bio, and workshop descriptions.

Think of some of your favorite brands or companies; Apple, YogaGlo, prAna, Clif Bar, Lululemon, and Wanderlust are a few popular ones among yoga teachers we've polled. These names come to mind because they have a clear, recognizable image associated with desirable qualities.

You may not know exactly how to turn the words and qualities you get from your own brand inquiry into your public face or brand. If you do have a good sense of graphic design and promotional writing, fantastic. If not, branding experts, graphic artists, and copywriters are in the business of turning your essence into a tangible presence. (If you reach out to them, consider offering to trade services with them.)

Know Your Target Market

Branding is as much about you as it is about the people who gravitate toward your style and brand identity. For example, because my brand is all about a caring approach to bringing ancient wisdom to modern yogis, along with a passion for environmental conservation, I tend to attract a target market of students who are seeking a yoga teacher they can believe in, one who cares about yoga's history and both its physical and its spiritual benefits. They see the bigger picture concerning health and whole living — mind, body, spirit — and they care about the world outside of themselves, the environment and the earth.

Once you've done the work to get to know yourself, the next step in developing your brand is to understand who the clients and yoga students are who will be attracted to your brand. If you don't know who your ideal client is, your marketing will be too broad to be effective. You need to make sure that what you're offering is a match for the audience that digs your teaching. If you do know your target market, it's much easier to build your brand identity. Knowing your students also allows you to offer a better product: your students will feel that your classes are customized especially for them. This cannot help but make them feel more fulfilled, happy, and accomplished in their practice. Giving your students what they want, helping them solve their problems and reach their goals, is like watching someone unwrap a present.

Knowing your ideal clients makes it easier to enjoy marketing and helps you succeed in attracting the kinds of students you love to spend time with. And teaching to people you resonate with is easier and more enjoyable.

To know and understand your students, you must see life through their eyes. Talk to them, ask them questions, listen to them, observe them, and compassionately put yourself into their shoes. Take the time to write down your thoughts about the qualities you want in your students.

The following exercise changed my entire way of teaching. It is partly this exercise that inspired me to create "90 Minutes to Change the World." Among other things, this exercise helped me understand what fellow teachers and teacher trainees might be seeking and how I could help them achieve their goals.

Answer the following questions for every kind of student or client you work with, including beginners, private clients, retreat clients, workshop students, group class students, and teacher trainees. If you run a studio, you can do the same thing.

Getting to Know Your Ideal Yoga Client

1. First, build a profile of your current yoga students.
    a. What are the demographics of your current students (age, occupation, income, marital status, kids)?
    b. List what you know about the "psychographics" of your students: their lifestyle, beliefs, values, interests, and hobbies.

2. Now consider the demographics and psychographics of your *ideal* students. Answer the following questions from the perspective of an ideal student, as though you are seeing the world as that student sees it.
    a. What is your biggest dream, vision, or goal with respect to relationships, health, career, family, and/or general mind-set?
    b. What is your biggest fear in developing a yoga practice?
    c. What are your favorite books, music, and TV shows?
    d. What magazines do you read?
    e. What blogs do you follow?
    f. What topics do you search for online?
    g. What conferences or events do you attend?
    h. What do you do in your free time?

      i.   What other teachers or experts do you already follow?

Analyze Your Data

Completing this questionnaire is creative and fun but also serious work. Take your time with the exercise. If you get hung up on a particular question, move on. Some of this sort of thinking about your students is natural and intuitive; you may already be doing it in the back of your mind. But it is still worth trying to clarify those thoughts and get them down in writing.

When you think about your students' dreams and ambitions, they may include things like "Have a fulfilled life," "Feel connected to family," "Have a sense of well-being," "Be loved," and "Feel empowered."

What are your ideal students' biggest fears or worst-case scenarios for practicing yoga? They might fear embarrassment, injury, being singled out as not good enough, feeling pain, or standing out as stiff or old. Can you offer these students coping skills, alignment techniques to help them open up, your empathy and compassion, practical props, modifications, or humor?

When I look at the lists of responses created by yoga teachers in my "90 Minutes" course, I see numerous class theme ideas, plus an abundance of material that can be used on flyers, in social media posts, blog articles, workshop descriptions, and in bios and website copy.

This exercise can provide valuable material that will help you relate to your ideal students and clients — right from the heart. It can inspire everything you do to present yourself, both in your classes and in your promotional work (your website, social media posts, biographical sketches, and so on). Your confidence and ability to deliver teaching that hits home for your students will also increase dramatically.

Do this exercise separately for every kind of teaching you undertake, such as retreats, workshops, series, group classes, or private lessons, and apply it to every aspect of your overall marketing plan.

The Five Ps of Marketing

As you begin to think about marketing your offerings, it's handy to consider what are classically called the five Ps:

1. *Product:* In all your offerings — including group classes, private lessons, retreats, and series — what services and/or products are you promoting, and what is their value to participants?
2. *Price:* Consider what the going rate for this product is in the area where it will be offered.
3. *Place:* Are you in a market or location that can support you as a yoga teacher? Do people in your location want what you have to offer?
4. *Promotion:* How will you get the word out about what you're offering?
5. *Position:* How is your product — teaching — positioned in the overall market? What other activities are competing for your potential students' time and attention? Is your target student choosing between yoga and Pilates, yoga and fitness, or yoga and something else? In my area (Boulder, Colorado), most potential students are choosing between yoga and outdoor activities, so I take that choice into account in my promotions and scheduling by emphasizing the therapeutic benefits of yoga to the athletic body and the fact that our events take place after the sun is down or on weekends, when people have more time.

Creating a Yoga Marketing Plan

Having defined your own goals and mission and identified the client group you want to reach, it's time to consider how you will reach them to promote your services and talents. A marketing plan does not have to be a long, formal document; nor is marketing something you do once and forget about. It is dynamic and needs regular planning and attention.

Devote some time to your marketing planning and efforts each day. For each special offering you have scheduled over the next year, consider the first three Ps (*product, price*, and *place*) and then come up with at least two or three actions you can take toward *promotion* of the event that take *position* into account. Every time you plan a new offering and add it to your schedule, repeat this process. Here's an example — my marketing plan for a recent arm balances workshop:

MARKETING PLAN

Product: Arm Balances Workshop
Price: $55
Place: 90 Monkeys, Boulder, CO
Position: Competing with Pilates and outdoor activities
Promotion: Execute the following marketing plan, chunk each task into a calendar, and set reminders

Website

Create event page on website (with ecommerce established)

Flyer or Postcard

Hire graphic designer and supply with content
Print 500 copies
Distribute in class and place in stores, gyms, coffee shops, etc., around town
Leave a stack at the workshop venue

Email

Mention in monthly newsletter for four months leading up to event
Send out a dedicated email about the workshop one month before event, one week before event, and the day before event if space still available

Announcements

Announce in all group classes and suggest to private clients

Facebook

Create event page and invite friends — use arm balance photo for the cover image
Post every other week and interact on the event page for three months prior, and then once a week in the last month before

event. Schedule posts ahead of time.
- Time marketing posts with arm balance photos for Facebook page on same day as all emails, and set a $100 budget for boosting posts
- If relevant and appropriate, post about the workshop in community Facebook groups

Twitter
- Post every other week for three months prior to event, and then once a week in the last month before event — use arm balance photo. Schedule posts ahead of time.

Instragram
- Post once a month in the three months prior to event and then every other week in the last month before event — use arm balance photo

Don't feel you have to ace marketing all in one day. Break it down into small steps and work at it consistently; schedule marketing work into your day so you don't feel overwhelmed. And remember that even one small effort — something like letting class members know about other classes you teach — can pay off.

Old-School Marketing: Alternatives to Social Networking

In the next chapter, we offer advice about using social media to your advantage, and for most yoga teachers, it's an integral part of their marketing efforts. But despite social media's growing dominance, it still makes sense to have supplementary offline marketing strategies, which can be very effective in getting the word out about your services.

Augmenting your social media strategy with some tried-and-true marketing methods to increase your exposure among your student base and colleagues is a sure way to be successful as a yoga teacher and reach all audiences where they dwell. Here are a few suggestions for more-traditional marketing:

- Advertise your services in the local community wellness publication(s). In many towns and cities, these kinds of publications serve as a directory for alternative health practitioners. They are usually found in stacks at health food stores, cafes, and bookstores.
- Leave your business card or postcard in coffee shops, health food stores, and other establishments popular with people likely to be interested in yoga. Spend some time thinking about this. If you teach a class for elders or pregnant women, don't just think about where to find them; also consider where you might reach their friends, family, and caregivers.
- Ask for referrals from existing students and private clients.
- Maintain a current email list of your students and use email newsletters to stay in touch.
- Attend the conferences on health, wellness, and self-actualization that come through town. Even though these events can feel huge and impersonal, they are places where you can connect with like-minded peers. I have met teachers who have influenced my work, vendors whose products I loved (and who might love my own future products!), and owners of retreat centers where I might teach. I've also had many conversations that have led to teaching invitations.
- If in-person networking makes you nervous, take a deep breath and introduce yourself to someone. Smile. Consider what it is they do, rather than what you do, and make a sincere comment, like "I love this aspect of your work," or ask, "How did you get into this work?" As the conversation progresses, you can find common ground to explain what you do. Your genuine interest or admiration should always be welcomed. If it isn't, that issue is most likely with them, not you.

CHAPTER SIX

Social Media

When I started teaching yoga, cell phones did not exist, let alone all the social media platforms available today. And given the speed at which these things seem to be moving, some of the platforms that are popular as I write — Facebook, LinkedIn, Twitter, and Instagram — may be passé when you read this book. In this chapter, I hope to offer advice that is valid for current social media platforms as well as for the new ones that are bound to come along.

Ironically, modern social networking is very much in line with yoga's centuries-old concept of connection, relationship, and union. Social networking brings people into dialogue across oceans. It lets big corporations communicate with far-flung customers, and it creates vibrant virtual communities. It offers forums where people can pour their hearts out, share their misfortunes, and ask for support in tough times. When tragedy strikes, such as the tsunami in Japan, Hurricane Sandy, or a school or workplace shooting, online communities mourn and take action together. Yet social media will only lean toward more positivity if we work to minimize the opportunistic, the unethical, and the predatory.

A WORD ABOUT EMAIL

Although social media platforms are leading to a drastic reduction in the use of email, it is unlikely to go away anytime soon. Marketing experts agree that building an email list is essential in any business. Having a substantial email list gives you a way to share your message, your offerings, and your services without having to compete with a torrent of posts on social platforms.

Why Bother?

Perhaps you feel that social networking will never be your thing, or perhaps you've tried it and, like many people, you're suffering from burnout from the endless feed of posts, tweets, and updates. The good news is that personal interaction will always remain an important way of letting people know about the good things you do. Indeed, face-to-face encounters are still the dominant source of word-of-mouth sharing, even more than online conversations.

That said, social media is also a form of word of mouth, but according to the book *Socialnomics* by Erik Qualman, it's word of mouth on steroids. He says, "Word of mouth is now *world* of mouth." While I used to tell yoga teachers that they could absolutely do fine without social media if they really wanted to remain offline, I've recently changed my tune. Today, 50 percent of the world's population is under thirty years old, and 96 percent of Millennials are on social media and would rather lose their sense of hearing than their technology!

This means that most of this huge number of potential yoga students have embraced social media as a way of life. According to Qualman, Facebook has so many users that its "population" is now larger than that of China. Instagram and Twitter are not far behind. It's become clear that social media is not a fad but the biggest thing to change society since the Industrial Revolution. Unless you specifically want to teach yoga to a more limited population, my suggestion is to jump in and embrace social media.

For yoga teachers, social media — whatever the platform — serves two vital functions:

1. *Communication:* Keeping a conversation going about yoga in between classes and establishing yourself as a thought leader in the yoga industry

2. *Marketing:* Helping students find you and engage with your teaching

Old-school methods like flyers and newsletters do the same things, but the newer platforms make it all happen faster and make it possible to reach more people than ever before. Social networking is just another channel by which to communicate.

On social media platforms, you can converse with your students. They can ask you questions between classes. You can see pictures of their children and the activities they enjoy, and they can learn more about you as well. All of this results in a richer, more dynamic — and ultimately more personal — connection between you and your students.

FEEL THE FEAR...AND DO IT ANYWAY

If you feel daunted by creating a presence on social media, ask yourself why. Is it because you lack technical skills, or because you feel you aren't worthy of being out there?

Or perhaps on some level you actually fear being successful? Maybe you aren't fully committed to being a yoga teacher or running a yoga business.

Strive to uncover the source of your fears. Bringing awareness to them is really the only way to get past them — and to claim your power to teach yoga successfully.

Many of us also suffer wounds to our self-esteem when our posts don't receive as many "likes" as we hoped, or our followers increase at a painfully slow rate, while our colleagues' seem to double in numbers every month. As with anything, if you become obsessive about numbers, you can lose sight of reality, which is this: you are a good person, you are a talented yoga teacher, you care about others, and you have much to offer, regardless of what your social media statistics look like! Take a deep breath and appreciate yourself from the deepest place of self-honor. Remember your greatness and your mission.

The Four Cs

Remember the five Ps of marketing in chapter 5: *product, price, place, promotion*, and *position*? Now marketers are embracing the four Cs of social media: *content, connecting, community*, and *curating*. Let's look at these in more detail.

Content

Sharing valuable content is the key to social media engagement. Is the content you are posting relevant to your target audience's interests, needs, and desires? What insights about yoga can you share with them?

Connecting

Have conversations, listen, and respond quickly to students' comments on social media. Your followers want to engage and learn from you, and when you nurture them, they are more likely to remain loyal to your brand.

To connect with your students, you also need to figure out which media platforms to use. Fortunately or unfortunately, yoga students tend to be on a variety of platforms. The most widely used are Facebook, Instagram, Twitter, and Snapchat, but specific categories of clients may be on different platforms, so you may have to manage multiple social media platforms. To find out who uses what, you can always survey your community!

Community

Social media provides community forums for both peer-to-peer communication and exchanges between peers and thought leaders. People look both to experts and to one another for help with their interests, issues, and needs. Creating forums for your students, whether via a Facebook group or a thread of comments on a blog, can be a great way to create and sustain a community around the practice.

Curating

With still images and video now dominating social media, it's becoming more and more important to curate content, almost like managing an art gallery. Instagram users, for example, work hard at presenting photos in their galleries that conform to a consistent type of photo or color palette. In addition to making sure your content is presented in an aesthetically appealing way, it's important to curate your posts for your distinct audience, so that the majority of posts are about sharing insights, useful information and links, and fun photos and videos rather than being strictly promotional.

Social Media Basics

When you're ready to dive in, consider taking an online social media course to sharpen your skills. I have used the social media courses offered on Coursera.com as a resource to stay current. Check out the latest trends and changes by reading current articles about the various platforms. Ask your peers, students, friends, and family about the networks they use and how they use them. Ask what kinds of posts they appreciate seeing and what rubs them the wrong way.

Here are a few tips for using social media platforms to get the most exposure for your content and business. We'll look at specific platforms in a moment, but these basic guidelines apply to using any social media platform:

- *Stay consistent.* If you venture online, stay active. Having an outdated or unused social networking account is like having an 800 number that no one answers. Set a regular schedule for posting on each platform that you know you can adhere to. If you can post three times a day on certain platforms, great. If you can't, pick a realistic schedule of days and times for posts to keep your followers engaged.
- *Keep your posts short.* Although lots of people still read long novels and magazine articles, we've come to expect online communications to be short and sweet. The phenomenon known as microblogging is common on Facebook and Instagram. Posts and photo captions become like tiny blogs.
- *Provide great content.* If you consistently provide useful and relevant content, whether it's your own material or shared from other

sources, your followers will look to you as a resource.
- *Curate your posts.* Post content that's consistent with your mission and core values. This will reinforce your brand over time.
- *Promote sparingly.* While it can be tempting to post only about your events and offerings, marketing posts do not receive as much engagement and can also cause people to unfollow you. On Facebook, for example, unengaging posts can also negatively affect your page's score in the Facebook algorithm, resulting in your post having little or no visibility in people's feeds. By contrast, your engaging content-oriented posts will keep your page's score high so that when you do market your offerings, people will actually see them!
- *Facilitate sharing.* Enable the Share buttons or set the defaults on your website and blog so that other people can pass along your content. Getting your posts and pictures shared, liked, retweeted, or repinned is the key to building your contacts. A bigger contact list helps you let more people know about the great work you do.
- *Have fun!* Social media is about networking and communication. If you're enthusiastic about engaging with your network, your posts will reflect it. This is your chance to spread your love of yoga.

Popular Social Media Platforms for Yogis

LinkedIn

LinkedIn is a site for professionals rather than purely for social networking. Having a detailed profile on LinkedIn is like having your best résumé online, accessible to those in your field at any time. If you want to be considered a yoga professional, no other networking site is more important. LinkedIn offers networking groups where yoga teachers can collaborate on professional matters. More important, it's a key site for contacting human resources managers to promote your workplace yoga offerings and for posting about the importance of yoga in the office.

Facebook

If you're comfortable with using Facebook and think it can help build your teaching career, we recommend creating a professional business page in addition to a personal profile.

To join Facebook, everyone has to create a personal profile page. This allows you to share details of your personal life with your Facebook friends. Who those friends are is up to you. Since you can have up to five thousand friends, many small business owners use their personal profile page for business as well, and add their clients as friends. However, this approach requires careful monitoring of what is posted there, by you or any of your friends. If someone shares those embarrassing pictures of your late-night dance party or your awful high-school yearbook photo, your yoga students can see them too! Therefore, it could be better to keep your personal profile page truly personal, friending only people who are real-life friends and family, not clients or friends of friends.

Because Facebook does not want you to use your personal profile page to market your business, the company has created special features for business use. A professional business page can have unlimited "likes" (or fans, as the feature was once called). Anyone who likes your page can see the content, so you need to be judicious about what you post there.

FACEBOOK TIPS

- Start "liking" other businesses' and colleagues' pages, especially those of businesses that serve an audience similar to yours.
- Check your news feed to see posts from the pages you like, and make a habit of commenting, liking, and sharing their content. This increases your visibility and means that followers of those pages may like your page, especially if you offer insight, humor, or helpful information in the comments.
- Create Facebook event pages to showcase your workshops, beginner series, retreats, and other offerings using the event page creator. Include all the specific details about the event and explain why people should attend. Event pages give people the chance to learn about the event and interact with other attendees. The sole disadvantage is that you can only invite your Facebook friends (meaning your personal page friends) individually to join the event.

Therefore to get the word out to your business page followers, you must post on your page or in relevant Facebook groups you belong to, asking people to visit the event page and RSVP if they plan to attend. Any posts made to an event page will pop up more reliably on the feeds of those who have been invited or have RSVP'd.

As you may have noticed, Facebook has changed its algorithm so that unless your post is organically engaging, it won't make it into people's feeds, to the dismay of many. As I mentioned, marketing posts generally are not as engaging as more personal content posts, and Facebook knows this. Therefore, they have forced businesses to boost their posts and pay to have them show up in people's feeds. This is why event pages are such a great workaround.

- Don't be shy. Nobody is being forced to look at your page, so you should never feel that you are being pushy or "spamming" other people. However, do be mindful of the fourth C of social media and *curate* your posts so that they emphasize content over promotion.

FACEBOOK AND ME

I was late to the game when I joined Facebook in 2009. The whole first month, I was a "lurker" because I was terrified of people seeing or interacting with me. Even though I was already known in the yoga world, I felt shy. This mode of communicating was new to me, and I was unsure of the consequences of posting or commenting. I was already inundated with emails and certainly didn't want more work.

I took baby steps to interact and found myself enjoying the connections with my students and others. Eventually, I started seeing a drop in the number of emails I was getting because I was communicating easily with lots of people on Facebook. It *is* a different way of connecting, often terser and more informal, but it is a connection, and it can be fun.

Instagram

You probably already know what Instagram does: it allows you to share photos and videos online and to dress them up by applying filters that give the images a look similar to old-school Polaroid images or photos from a Kodak Instamatic film camera, as well as offering all the modern features of the best photo apps. You can use a variety of hashtags to categorize the images so that they will come up in viewers' searches.

This highly visual social media platform has become hugely popular with yoga enthusiasts. It abounds with pictures of creative evolutions of ever more advanced asanas, sent in from yogis all over the world. Instagram offers a fine example of the pros and cons of online promotion. Viewers might ask, "What's with all these incredibly advanced yoga selfies?" or "Can I do yoga without doing *that*?"

So how can you use Instagram for a yoga business? The key is to use images to tell a story — about what you teach and who you are, about your brand and the people or studios you work with. Think like your client. What can a photograph tell them about your services?

INSTAGRAM TIPS

- Show pictures of the studios where you work.
- Give viewers a backstage pass. For example, take a picture of the books you have open when you're preparing for class, your notebook with stick-figure drawings of the class, and your feet sitting in sukasana on your mat as you're doing all this.
- Document a day of teaching yoga and include students in the photos. (Be sure to get the students' explicit consent before posting their photos.)
- When you travel, especially for yoga training, workshops, or retreats, share photos from the start of the trip to the end. Take your online audience along!
- Use relevant, specific hashtags. Research hashtags that are trending (meaning popular at the moment, yielding numerous images in a search) and use them in relevant photos.

A WORD ON SOCIAL MEDIA YOGA FAME

While this book was being written, a new phenomenon in the yoga world emerged: the "Insta-famous yogi" or Instagram yogis. Yoga hobbyists, new yoga teachers, and veteran teachers alike have jumped on the Instagram bandwagon, posting photos and videos of their practice — each one more bendy and acrobatic than the next. The imagery is artistic and often shot with beautiful backdrops, such as beaches with cerulean blue water, mountaintops, and dramatic urban landscapes.

On the plus side, all this yoga sharing has brought the global yoga community together, friendships have been forged in real life, and many people have decided to try yoga for the first time after being inspired by these posts. On face value it offers a platform to share ideals, values, and lessons in life.

Like many using Instagram, yogis are taking advantage of the plethora of filtering apps available that not only help make their photos pop aesthetically but also can smooth skin, whiten teeth, and reshape body parts. The less you wear, and the deeper you bend, the more followers and more fame you might have.

Brands hoping to break into the yoga world are willing to pay yogis with large accounts to post about their products. A few yoga teachers are even earning more through endorsements on Instagram than they are from teaching, resulting in some controversy! Are the teachers merely selling ad space on their accounts, or are they endorsing products they truly believe in sharing?

A more global concern is how social media fame is impacting the yoga world, in particular *studentship* among yogis. Impressionable yogis are starting to confuse fame and big followings for excellence in yoga and yoga teaching. "Insta-fame" is not necessarily the equivalent of being well educated, seasoned, wise, accomplished, or professional, and it's not a substitute for the years of study, perseverance, and patience it takes to be a yogi. You can only be as good a teacher as you are a student.

Twitter

Anyone who uses Twitter regularly will tell you that its power lies not so much in its content as in its ability to connect you to other people. Currently limited to 140 characters, Twitter communications (tweets) are very straightforward and simple.

The real power of Twitter for business promotion lies in getting other people to pick up on and share (retweet) what you say with their followers. For example, say you post an insight about yoga, and someone with a sizeable Twitter following reads and retweets it. That means your tweet was exposed not only to your regular followers, but to this other person's Twitter network as well. The more this happens, the more exposure your tweet will get, and the more people will want to follow you on Twitter. The power of this is exponential.

Think of Twitter less as a popularity contest and more as a business tool. You have something to offer. More people benefit from your offering if your Twitter following grows. Remember, too, that Twitter communications are read by people who have opted in. Therefore these people want to be in contact with you.

TWITTER TIPS

- Pick a simple, short user name that will become your Twitter "handle." Use your real name if possible.
- Use the List function to view the tweets from people and organizations that matter most to you. Include those who produce useful content, friends, family, local yoga colleagues, teachers, and companies you like, but be selective, otherwise the "noise" on your main stream can be overwhelming.
- The maximum number of characters in a tweet is 140. However, it's good to limit your tweets to 120 characters, leaving 20 characters available for people to use when they retweet the message. Edit your tweets carefully to make them into powerful little nuggets of goodness.
- When sharing URL links, use a service like Bitly.com to shorten long links to 20 characters. This gives you 100 characters to write

about the content of that link.
- Tweet compelling content that's relevant to your target audience.
- Share snapshots of what is happening in your life right now to give your audience a window into your everyday experience.
- Every Twitter follower wants to be nurtured. Stay in touch with your followers by consistently providing them with valuable information, and offer advice and encouragement. Doing so establishes you as an expert in your field. Responding to people's direct messages and @ mentions reminds your Twitter followers that there is a real person behind the Twitter handle available to give them assistance, advice, and support and answer questions about events. As you gain more followers, it may be difficult to answer every tweet, but setting aside some time to get to as many as possible will help you retain the followers you have.
- Check your mentions feed regularly to see when people have sent you a tweet or mentioned you in a tweet. Write back to anyone who mentions you and thank them, and give yoga advice if asked.
- Twitter's search feature is your friend. The search box is at the top of the screen on Twitter.com. Use searches for yoga-related keywords to find and start interacting with new tweeters. You'll make friends fast, and some connections might lead to great opportunities! All it takes is one reply that you can compose in less than thirty seconds.
- If you use Twitter extensively, we highly recommend using a desktop client like Hootsuite or Buffer to help optimize and schedule your tweets.
- Remember, the more you retweet (RT) other tweeters' content, the more you in turn will get retweeted, which expands your reach far beyond your own followers.

I was about to start writing about Pinterest, essentially a giant online bulletin board where you can "pin" and share images that interest you, and Snapchat, a video messaging app, but I realized that if I kept writing about different social media platforms, this chapter would go on forever. So let's stop here and return to general social media advice that you can adapt to any new platform that comes along.

Being Personal in Your Professional Posts

Social media has changed the way we present ourselves professionally. Prospective students now expect to be able to check out a yoga teacher online, through tweets or Facebook status updates, before even attending a class. While you might feel uncomfortable about airing parts of your personal life online in this way, it's part of doing business today. In my public posts, I certainly don't put any words or photos out there that I'd regret, but I do share snippets of who I am, what interests me, and what I think might inspire my readers. For example, on the next page is a post I made on Instagram about how my practice had evolved in recent years. Even though it wasn't a professional photograph, the post was personal and honest, so it received more engagement than other, less-personal posts.

Because social media is interactive and is a two-way exchange, it also offers ways to gain valuable information and feedback. Clients and customers have easy and open methods of sharing positive feedback and gratitude, whether it's a "like" on Facebook or a detailed five-star review. On the other hand, of course, businesses are also much more vulnerable to negative feedback and even harassment from dissatisfied clients, competitors, or random "haters." There is a new level of transparency — and thus vulnerability — for even small businesses today. Businesses and even yoga teachers need to have strategies and methods for handling dissatisfied clients gracefully and openly.

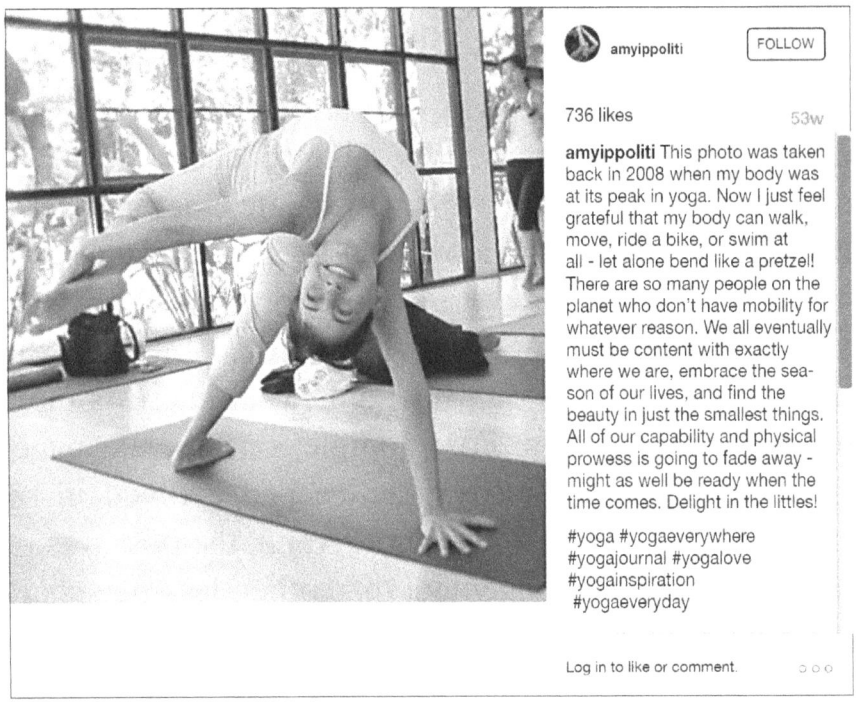

RESPONDING TO HATERS

If you discover that someone has posted a negative comment about you or your teaching on a social media platform, here's an approach for responding to and defusing it professionally.

1. *Acknowledge* the commenter's point as important and welcomed. Be gracious.
2. *Respond* to the comment. If the person has misunderstood or misrepresented your position on something, politely correct the error. If the comment makes a valid point, acknowledge it and apologize if necessary. If you feel that there is a genuine difference of opinion, or you don't want to prolong an argument, you may suggest that you both agree to disagree.
3. *Wish the commenter well*. Be kind and friendly as you close your reply. Resist the temptation to tell the person off or say something like, "If you don't like what I post, then unfollow me!" To me, that approach is dismissive rather than engaging and does not embrace this person's right to speak and be

heard. A calm, centered, and peace-loving reply will win you the support of other readers, whereas a lashing out or a rebuttal would inevitably result in unfollowers.

A student who came to a retreat with me had this printed on her T-shirt: "May your life someday be as awesome as you pretend it is on Facebook." I had to stop the class to read it and laugh.

Deciding what to share, and how to present it on social media platforms can be tricky. It's easy to portray an "awesome" life, and, as the T-shirt slogan suggests, there's a lot of pressure to show that your life is just as awesome as everyone else's. But in addition to not being honest, being relentlessly upbeat and self-promotional doesn't foster genuine connection. (Nor does a self-absorbed oversharing of personal details.) Be yourself.

Although many people choose not to disclose personal details in social media profiles, I believe in using my own name and using a close head shot as my profile picture. Transparency isn't difficult when we aren't pretending.

Overall, always strive to be genuine — about who you are, what you offer, and why you do what you do. And remember that you need never share or reveal more than you are comfortable with. You can't go wrong with these guidelines as your foundation.

CHAPTER SEVEN

Forming Good Professional Relationships

As yoga teachers, we are in a relationship business. To be successful, we must embrace relationship building on many different levels. It's especially important for us to see our students not as devotees who should serve their teacher or guru but as paying clients deserving of nurturing care and attention.

There are seven primary kinds of relationships that are important to yoga teaching:

1. Relationship with the divine
2. Relationship with oneself
3. Relationships with family and friends
4. Relationships with individual students
5. Relationships with staff and colleagues
6. Online relationships
7. Relationships with classes and community

For your own personal growth and for the good of your teaching, it's important to assess each of these types of relationships in your life and ask yourself whether any of them need more attention. This may seem repetitive, but self-inquiry and growth are a huge part of being a yogi.

Let's consider some of these relationships in more detail.

Relationship with the Divine

When we are connected to the divine, we feel more inspired, and thus we teach at our best. But this relationship often gets put on hold when we get busy. Today, with all the distractions of electronic devices and social media, it has become more and more challenging to unplug and find a moment of quiet. When I feel cut off from spirit, I increase my meditation and mantra repetition, get outside, put my bare feet in the grass, light a candle, or write in a gratitude journal. It does not take much to revive the dialogue.

Relationship with Oneself

Yoga teachers are taught to model self-care, but they're often not consistent about following through. Being more stressed than your students is not a basis for good teaching. One of our graduates reported that after she consciously increased her self-care and spent more time unplugged, her teaching improved dramatically. Her students noticed and responded very positively to the difference. We look at self-care at greater length in chapter 11.

Relationships with Family and Friends

According to the author and actor Ben Stein, "Personal relationships are the fertile soil from which all advancement, all success, all achievement in real life grows." Your closest friends, loved ones, and family are vital to your growth and ability to stay inspired as a yoga teacher. When these relationships are nurtured, you also model the importance of personal relationships to your students.

To make sure you're devoting time to tending these relationships, schedule a regular date night with your partner, put regular hang-out time with your kids on your calendar, keep in touch with out-of-town family more consistently, or set up frequent get-togethers with friends.

Relationships with Individual Students

Early in my career, more than a decade ago, I taught a weekly class in a basement room to sixty-five wholehearted New Yorkers at Crunch Fitness in Manhattan. Little did I know that the relationships I formed in that gym would lead to meaningful lifelong connections.

Every week, I came to class early and stayed after to talk with students, work on their therapeutic issues and injuries, answer their questions — and just hang out and gab. Some people sat around talking for an hour afterward. Most nights after class I brought students with me upstairs to Jivamukti Yoga Center to catch the tail end of Krishna Das's weekly New York kirtans. We'd sing and sway, do *puja*, and delight in the fruit salad prasad.

I am still in touch with many students from that time. Some of them went on to travel with me to new and beautiful places on retreat, and some became master yoga instructors in their own right.

These kinds of students can become loyal supporters who spread the word about your classes and help build a loving community of people around a common interest: yoga.

Relationships with Staff and Colleagues

Do you make a habit of being kind and speaking respectfully to gym and studio staff? I don't claim to be any kind of saint, but I do my best to be friendly and considerate to these colleagues. Not only is this important to my sense of myself, but it makes for easier and more collegial working relationships, which make for better teaching.

Stories abound of yoga teachers at fitness gyms who act entitled, elitist, and pretentious, brusquely demanding specific conditions for their classes and acting as if the other gym staff are ignorant about yoga in general. How much cooperation do you think these teachers are likely to receive?

Because yogis often practice in community, we have a tendency to develop what I call yoga tunnel vision. Yoga, like anything else, can be taken to fanatical levels, to the point where practitioners can't relate to non-yogis! And isn't yoga supposed to be about connection?

Good manners, curiosity, kindness, helpfulness, generosity, enthusiasm, and sensitivity go a long way to demonstrate the spiritual and emotional benefits of yoga, as well as the physical ones, and help yoga continue to grow in the mainstream. Here are some specific ways to nurture relationships with colleagues at a gym or studio.

- *Get to know other teachers at the gym or studio and take their classes.* Learning from other yoga teachers is a vital part of a yoga practice. Taking fitness classes at the gym can boost other aspects of your physical health as well as help you develop good relationships with the other instructors.
- *Attend all meetings and social functions of the gym or studio.* Showing up for meetings and gatherings where you work, even if you are busy, does two very important things: it helps you know and be a part of the team, and it increases your visibility among managers and students. Managers who see you getting involved with the gym or studio are more likely to give your name when a student asks what class to take or is looking for a teacher to work at a special function, like a wedding party. Attending studio functions lets you get to know current students and gets your name out among potential new students.
- *Keep lines of communication open with colleagues and staff.* Whether you're a studio owner/manager or an employee, touch base regularly with the people you work alongside. Share your needs, goals, visions, feedback, and even grievances. Don't let ill-feeling fester to the point where neither party is willing to try to resolve a problem.
- *Maintain good communication by establishing it* before *there's a problem.* If you teach at a studio, for example, chat with the studio owners about getting classes covered, or share with them how you handled a difficult student. By establishing a dialogue when nothing is wrong, you will have a good channel of communication in place if you need to bring up a touchy subject.
- *Be friendly with teachers of other styles of yoga.* It's simply unattractive when a yoga teacher says something negative about another teacher or style of yoga. Don't do it. You're the one who ends up looking bad. Instead, use differences in opinion as an opportunity to see and learn from another perspective.
- *When you don't like something, offer a solution.* If you are upset about something going on where you work, go directly to the source or the person in charge, state the problem, and then offer to find a solution. This way you won't be seen as a gossiper or complainer.

- *Be a "go-giver," not a "go-getter."* A go-getter comes in, teaches a class, and leaves. A go-giver comes in, sees what he can do to pitch in, and asks what announcements need to be made for upcoming events. After class, he folds blankets, puts away props, blows out candles, and picks up water bottles and Kleenex left behind.

  Never think that you are above these tasks. Making this effort increases the feeling of goodwill in the studio, and studio managers who see you pitching in will be more apt to give you prime teaching slots when they open up.

CHAPTER EIGHT

Managing Your Business Finances

Whether we like it or not, dealing with finances is an inevitable part of working as a yoga teacher. Fortunately, we can learn to do it in ways that reflect our values and visions. We can manage the financial aspects of our business well so that we can pay our bills, live our lives without worry, and build a successful business that enables us to share yoga's benefits and live according to our beliefs and values.

Being stressed out about money will affect your teaching, consciously or unconsciously. Money troubles can make you unfocused and stressed, worrying about how many students are in the room instead of quality teaching. Taking on more classes than you can easily manage in order to make ends meet can make you scattered and unorganized in the classroom. Finally, fretting about money robs teaching of its joy, and your self-esteem will suffer if you come to believe it's impossible for you to make a living.

This chapter takes you through a number of strategies for managing your business finances. You may feel you cannot afford to spend time or money on these financial services or tasks. However, we have found that most yoga teachers who are doing well invested in their future by having a sound financial system in place before they began making substantial money. Let's start with the basics.

- *Create a financial team.* This ideally includes a bookkeeper, an accountant, and/or a financial adviser.

- *Set up a business entity.* Although you can teach yoga and accept payment under your own name, your personal financial situation and your long-term business plans may make it advisable to create a separate business entity. In the United States, you have several options for doing so, and an experienced tax adviser or accountant can help you decide which would be best.
- *Create a bank account just for your yoga teaching and business.* Many yoga teachers simply put the money they make from teaching into a personal account, but if you are going to honor your teaching and take your business seriously, it is important to have clear boundaries. One way to do this is by having a separate account for your business. Talk to your financial advisers about the best way to set up the account.
- *Pay yourself first!* From all my business reading and the many conversations I've had with health and wellness entrepreneurs, it is clear that most successful people pay themselves first. This doesn't necessarily mean literally cutting yourself a paycheck: it means treating a designated portion of your business income as fair payment for your own hard work. Of course, if you run a studio or hire other staff, you need to budget for rent, wages, and other expenses, but this doesn't mean that you should underpay yourself.
- *Save a little every month.* A key part of paying yourself first is investing in yourself by saving. Seeing money grow in a savings or investment account is very rewarding. As your money increases, so does your confidence! The best way to get into the habit of saving is to set up automatic payments into your savings account.

　　As a starting point, I suggest putting at least 10 percent of your teaching income into savings. This may seem like a daunting amount to set aside when you have bills to pay. But, again, this is a strategy used by many successful teachers and leaders, even when they were first starting out. I have found that once you've put money aside for yourself, you always find a way to earn the amount you need to cover the bills. All the practices outlined in this book are designed to help you increase your earnings, so have faith in yourself!

Insurance

Yoga teachers need two kinds of insurance: health insurance for themselves and their dependents, and liability insurance to protect them against any mishaps that may occur in classes.

Health Insurance

If you live in a country where health care is subsidized and you are already covered, count your blessings and skip ahead! If you live in the United States, read on.

I was shocked to learn how many yoga teachers do not have health insurance in the United States because they feel they cannot afford the monthly premiums. Practicing yoga and living a healthy lifestyle may help ward off illness, but there are no guarantees. At the risk of sounding like a mom, what would you do if you got into a car accident and couldn't pay your hospital bills? Have you ever seen announcements for medical fund-raisers in the yoga community? These are typically held to raise funds for a yoga teacher who could not afford medical bills because he or she did not have health insurance.

Depending on where you live in the United States, you may be able to find a health insurance plan with affordable premiums through the Affordable Health Care Act ("Obamacare"). If money is really tight, get a policy that covers you just for catastrophic health events. You'll find a way to pay the premium.

If you already have health insurance, make sure you fully understand the kind of policy you have and double-check exactly what you are covered for. For example, a friend of mine, a personal trainer, had a snowmobile crash. His hospital stay cost a fortune. Although his health insurance policy offered comprehensive benefits, he had failed to notice that it did not cover this kind of incident. Because his work, like teaching yoga, was hands-on and physical, he could not return to work to pay the bills. He lost everything. Don't place yourself at this kind of risk: put the money aside for a health insurance policy and read all the fine print.

Liability Insurance

Most of us don't want to believe that our students would ever be litigious, and in truth, most students are not. Moreover, when properly taught, yoga is a very safe form of physical activity. Occasionally, however, yoga teachers face liability lawsuits. In 2009, a student sued a prominent yoga studio in Boulder, Colorado. The student claimed that he had been permanently injured by a hands-on adjustment given by one of the teachers. The studio and teacher were protected from financial disaster by their liability insurance. Paying for liability insurance is very inexpensive compared to unconsciously worrying about injuries every time you teach or having a potentially devastating lawsuit hanging over you.

Business liability insurance is available from various sources. *Yoga Journal* works with a great insurance company to provide a liability policy called Yoga Journal Teachers Plus that costs, as I write, under $200 a year.

LIABILITY RELEASES

Yoga studios generally require all new students to sign a liability release form, or waiver. If you are conducting yoga classes outside of an established studio, however, it's your responsibility to have students release you from liability. It's best to consult with an attorney to create a standard liability release you can have students sign to protect you, in addition to carrying your own liability insurance policy.

Contribution and *Seva*

Does the topic of charitable contributions belong in a chapter on business finances? For yoga teachers, yes. Involvement in volunteer work, charity, philanthropy, or *seva* (the Sanskrit word for service) is a huge part of what yoga is about — and, as an added bonus, it inspires your teaching. The beauty of service is that it not only assists the people you are serving but also enhances your self-esteem, and this makes you a better teacher. Here are just a few of the many benefits of being involved in some form of *seva:*

- It teaches humility
- It inspires and gives your identity as a teacher more meaning
- It is a great way to build community and connection
- It gives your teaching more purpose
- It cultivates abundance and energy, because the universe sees that you are giving back and that you are ready for more
- It makes you feel uplifted because you feel useful

Giving back is fundamental to human existence. For most of the last month of my grandmother's life, when she was in hospice, she would hug and give everyone sweet compliments. It was her way of giving back, even though she was weak and in pain. When she reached a point where she could barely talk or wrap her arms around people anymore I saw that she was getting ready to leave. It was as though if she could no longer give back, she was done. She lived only another three days.

Being of service to others helps us feel useful and valued. Having *seva* as part of our lives can be a source of deep motivation and inspiration. It also makes for wonderful anecdotes to share with our students. When we give and we feel of use, not only in our teaching but in other ways too, we can share our feelings of encouragement and inspiration with our students.

Part III

TEACHING WELL

CHAPTER NINE

Class Planning and Preparation

To teach well, we all need a good "container." The Sanskrit word for container is *dharana*. The container holds what you put into it. Having excellent training and being a skilled teacher are important things to put into your container, but solid preparation and organization also need to be in there.

It's easy to understand why students appreciate good preparation. Teachers who are well organized remember what they did in the previous class, continue where they left off, and know and remember the health concerns or challenges of regular students. Their classes flow well, with smooth sequences, helpful cues, and interesting themes and anecdotes. And organization gives the teachers themselves the mental space to plan classes that keep things fresh for them as well as for their students.

Yet in a recent poll of our teacher trainees, Taro and I found that only 22 percent always felt prepared and organized for class. What are the challenges that keep us from preparing well? Here are some suggestions to identify and help overcome them.

Create a Packing List

Create a list of things you'll need for each day's classes, and consult it before you leave home so that you won't forget any important items. My list includes items I need for teaching, such as my class plans or binder, music, bells (to take students out of savasana), and yoga mat and cushion, if needed. Sometimes I remind myself to bring along a handout or small gift for the students too. I also include marketing materials, such as my mailing list sign-up sheet, postcards for upcoming events, and business cards. Making a list might sound trivial; however, there's a reason pilots go through a preflight checklist no matter how often they fly. How many times have you gone to a grocery store to pick up three items, only to return home with ten items and only one of the three you intended to buy?

Keep a Teaching Binder

I love my teaching binder because it helps me keep my teaching fresh and inspired. Your binder is where you can store all your ideas, teaching notes, stick-figure drawings, client notes, theme ideas, and thoughts about yoga philosophy and life in general.

You can create a tool like this either in an old-style three-ring binder or on an electronic device. Either way, it should be in a form you can bring with you and refer to easily in class. I still use a pen and paper, because they somehow slow me down and get me back to basics. Even if you're a devoted tablet or computer user, you might try writing by hand once in a while to see if it provokes a different line of thought.

Having a binder keeps all your ideas at your fingertips. On days when you are not feeling inspired, you can open the binder and get an idea for class.

I suggest keeping the following sections in your binder.

Mission Statement

Your mission statement comes first and foremost in your binder (see page 35). In this section you can keep all your brainstorming notes. I can't tell you how many times I have felt dull and uninspired before teaching a class. When I ask myself, "Why am I doing this?" and look at my mission statement, I always get a spark of inspiration and an idea for the class.

Values

Keep the list of values that you came up with earlier (see page 29) in this section so you have it at your fingertips.

REHEARSALS

If you teach a style of yoga in which you typically share more than simple physical instructions — for example, when you are working with a theme or integrating yoga philosophy — what you share has to be genuine, concise, and easy for students to relate to so that it doesn't come across as pretentious or hokey. If you rehearse what you plan to say to a friend or significant other before class and accept feedback, it will come across much more effectively and genuinely.

Contemplations and Anecdotes

One of the things that makes a yoga class different from a fitness class is that it often includes an inspirational message given at the beginning of or during class. Students often enjoy hearing teachers' personal stories or their takes on subjects such as the *yamas* and *niyamas*, the *gunas*, or the *koshas*. It's critical, though, to keep these messages succinct, sincere, and focused, or they'll irritate students instead of inspiring them. Regularly write down the insights and metaphors that occur to you and collect them in your binder. Consulting this treasure trove before or during class can help you frame an effective message that's uniquely yours.

Themes

In this section you can keep an ongoing list of ideas for class themes (see the next chapter for details). Browsing the list is a great way to come up with an idea for your next class.

Class Plans

Keeping your class plans all in one place gives you flexibility: you can reuse a class plan on a day when you don't have time to plan anything new, or reuse a successful plan with a different group of students. The more you plan your classes, the more plans you'll have to draw on for future use. See my example of a class planning template later in this chapter.

Keeping a library of plans also serves as a great record of what you have done previously with your students. It's also a good place to note sequences you enjoyed while taking classes from other teachers.

If you are auditioning to teach somewhere new, or anytime you are nervous, use your favorite plans (the classes where you knocked it out of the park) to boost your confidence and offer your best teaching.

REPETITION IS THE MOTHER OF LEARNING

Some teachers feel they are cheating or lazy if they repeat a class plan. While it's important to be fresh and do different things with your students, a certain amount of repetition is appropriate. In fact, many students love repetition and the chance to improve on something they have done before. Yoga is a *practice*, after all!

Cues and Instructions

Knowing your poses and demonstrating them perfectly is not the same thing as being able to explain them clearly to students during class when you are not in the pose. If you write up your cues and instructions, you can work through them and rehearse them before class. After class, you can come back and record the cues that worked best for students.

If you teach vinyasa yoga and are new to teaching, this can be a place to get clear on inhale versus exhale instructions. When I first had to teach a sun salutation, I could not remember how to connect the elements of the sequence to inhalation and exhalation. So I wrote out my cues for the sequence of a sun salutation word for word and practiced with a tape recorder before I taught.

If you use technical instructions or cues based on anatomical alignment, or if you tend to confuse left and right, working the cues out on paper helps you say them clearly and precisely. Teachers who can provide succinct instructions to help their students get into the correct poses provide a much smoother class experience.

DO THE TWIST

The instructions for getting students into a simple twist like ardha matsyendrasana can be very complex. To illustrate this point, compare these two sets of placement instructions.

1. "Okay. What we're going to do now is cross your right leg over the left knee and place that foot on the ground. Then bend that left knee so your foot sits by your hip — I mean the right hip. Sit up tall, and then twist to your right, placing your right hand on the ground behind you and wedging your left elbow against the left-hand side of your left knee — oh, wait, I meant the right knee. Inhaling, straighten your spine, and exhaling, twist to your right and look to the right."
2. "Cross your right foot over your left knee and place it on the floor. Bend your left leg and draw the heel toward your right hip. Hook your left elbow to the outside of your right knee and place your right hand behind you. As you inhale, get tall. As you exhale, twist to the right and look over your right shoulder."

Which one did you understand better? The second one was written out ahead of time and is clear, short, and succinct.

Vinyasa Flows

A variety of mini-vinyasa flows (shorter sequences within the overall class sequence) helps keep classes interesting. Anyone can come up with new sequences using a sticky mat as a laboratory. Trying them out first instead of inventing them on the fly in class will allow you to make sure that they're accessible and graceful before springing them on your students.

Creative mini-vinyasas are like gold! Write them down and file them in this section.

Quotes

Keep a section of your favorite quotations by famous authors, teachers, and artists and use them to support your class themes and inspire your students with something more than just stretching.

You can also file quotes according to topic, such as self-love, getting through difficult times, seeing the silver lining, empowerment, and mindfulness. Then if you are teaching a class on any of these themes, you can easily find appropriate quotes to use in class.

Student and Client Notes

Keep a record of your clients' achievements, challenges, and poses done in class. This is useful for group classes, but it's especially good for private clients, because usually more time passes between private sessions, and it's easy to forget what you covered in the previous session.

Useful Verbs

All yoga cues use verbs, both literal and metaphorical. Words and phrases like *extend, root, ground, draw in, reach out*, and *melt* are used to describe movement in yoga.

It's easy to fall into a stale pattern of repeating the same verbs over and over. Keep a list of good alternatives for describing poses and sequences, drawn from your reading, other classes and activities, and even the thesaurus.

Four categories of verbs are particularly relevant to yoga sequences. Here are some you can use to give students a richer experience.

General: Words and phrases like *ground, extend, expand, inflate, widen, tap into, attract*.

Hydraulic: When you are teaching a class that has a theme relating to the water element, you can use verbs such as *pour, stream*, and *flow*.

Photic: For any class theme that has to do with light — finding your inner light, finding the light at the end of the tunnel, or being a brighter light in the world — consider using verbs such as *shine, beam, radiate, blaze, glow*, and *sparkle*.

Sonic: In a class with a theme related to vibration or pulsation, use verbs related to sound, such as *echo, resonate*, and *reverberate*.

How Much Should You Plan?

How structured should your classes be? Should you adhere to a rigid class plan or suit your sequences to your own state of mind, the vibe among the students in the room, or sudden inspiration? Here are issues to consider on both sides.

Pros of Planning

Planning is calming and gives you confidence, especially when you are starting out. The process helps you get to know your material, thus increasing the capacity of your *dharana!* Students appreciate that you have taken the time to think about the class beforehand. And even if you want to take a more fluid and improvisational approach in class, it helps to have a backup plan. It can give you the confidence to experiment, knowing that if inspiration fails, you can always return to the plan.

Cons of Planning

Sticking too closely to a class plan can make your teaching overly rigid and can make it harder for you to be present to the students in the room and what is needed in the moment. It can close you off from other possibilities and make you unspontaneous.

There are ways to strike a balance between rigid planning and chaos. Although I recommend that you always have some kind of plan, I also think that good, deep preparation for teaching should enable you to depart from that plan when the occasion arises. As you teach, pay attention to what's happening in the room rather than always adhering to your plan.

Be confident in your teaching. The fact that you have invested the time and thought to plan a class means that you have all the skills and knowledge in your head to teach without notes.

Use a Class Planning Template

Using a template to plan allows you to consider all the elements of your yoga class beforehand, including your theme, your sequence of poses, adjustments you want to offer, music you might want to play, and how to pace the class.

Once you have planned about twenty classes using a template, you'll have a valuable repertoire of class plans that you can reuse or adapt. This can be especially useful if you're short on time to plan a class or if you have to change a plan on the fly to meet the specific needs of the students who showed up. Even after all my years of teaching, I still use my class planning templates.

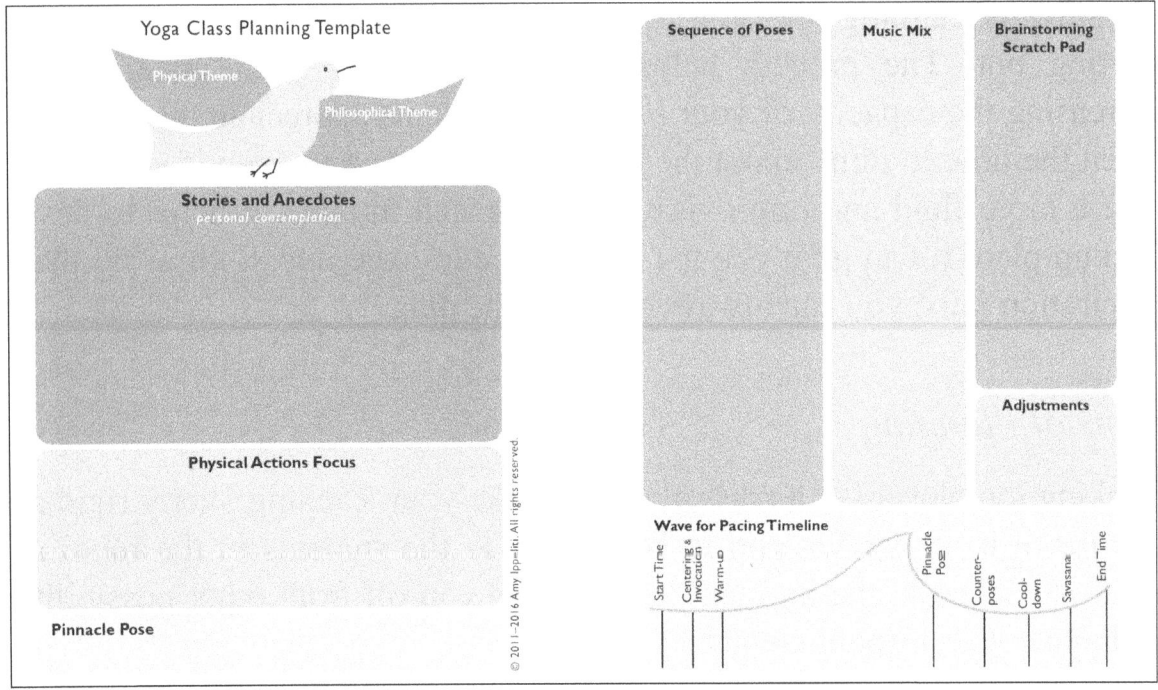

The template shown here (adjusted slightly to fit the pages of this book) is the result of years of scribbling down sequences, contemplations, and pacing notes for my classes. I wanted a structure that would let me write down all the elements of a good yoga class. After working on a number of iterations, I presented my design to a graphic artist, who came up with the template I still use today. You can use it as a model to create your own template, or find a downloadable version at 90Monkeys.com.

The template includes two visual elements: the bird at the top, to reflect the class theme; and the wave at the bottom, to illustrate the timing and flow of the class.

I usually start planning by choosing a theme, either physical or philosophical. If I'm choosing a physical theme, I ask myself what physical actions I want to focus on in the class. What is the pinnacle pose I want the class sequences to build toward? If I'm using a philosophical theme, I ask myself what the philosophical message of the class will be. There's more information on themes later in this chapter. Once you've chosen a theme, work through the different boxes on the template:

- Use the "Brainstorming Scratch Pad" box to jot down thoughts and ideas about any aspects of the class before you organize them into the template. Of course, you can also do this on a separate sheet of paper.
- In the "Stories and Anecdotes" box, note a source of inspiration, such as a personal story, quote, or current event. Relate this source of inspiration to the students' lives.
- In the "Pinnacle Pose" box, choose a pinnacle or apex pose that corresponds to the physical actions and philosophical theme. It should be the most challenging pose of the class and of appropriate difficulty for the majority of the students. (This step is optional, as you can teach a perfectly great class that never peaks to a particular pose.)
- In the "Physical Actions Focus" box, reflect on key physical actions you want to focus on, such as those required for the pinnacle pose (if any), or how the physical actions of the class relate to the philosophical theme.

- In the "Sequence of Poses" box, write out your full class sequence of poses.
- In the "Music Mix" box, if you plan to use music, write out your full playlist here, corresponding with the sequence. If you don't use music, you can leave this blank.
- In the "Adjustments" box, write out any key hands-on adjustments you'd like to offer your students that might be relevant given the pose sequence.
- Use the wave graphic to map out the amount of time you want to spend on each element of the class. Mark the class's start and end times at the two ends of the wave, and work inward from there, writing down the target time for starting each element of the class.

STANDARD SEQUENCING ELEMENTS OF AN ASANA CLASS

Every teacher has a slightly different take on sequencing, but in general you want to include and time the following elements:

Centering: Centering helps students transition to the practice from their busy days.

Warm-up: A warm-up eases students into their bodies before they perform any challenging poses.

Standing poses: Standing poses work well in the first half of class because they warm up the body so effectively. They are a classic way to teach alignment techniques and build stamina and confidence.

Abdominals or core work: Engaging the core happens naturally throughout the practice; however, it can be useful to teach specific core or "ab" work to prepare and strengthen the body for the increased range of motion and flexibility required for most bendy yoga poses.

Inversions and arm balances: Like core work and standing poses, inversions and arm balances demand stamina, build heat, and engage the core, so they are great for strengthening the body before moving on to poses that demand flexibility.

Preparatory poses: Before attempting more advanced or pinnacle poses, lead students through a series of poses to warm up and target the specific body parts involved.

Pinnacle pose or more challenging asanas: Using the wave, budget enough time for students to experiment and play with the pinnacle pose or the grouping of challenging asanas.

Counterposes: After the pinnacle pose or set of challenging asanas, it's time to teach a series of counterposes that counteracts the movements performed during the peak of the class.

Cool-down/seated poses: As part of the cool-down period, it's nice to add seated poses, such as hip openers and forward bends, before going into the stillness of savasana.

Meditation: You may choose to add a brief meditation period where students can sit, close their eyes, and take in and feel the practice in silence.

Savasana (final relaxation): Working backward from the tail end of the wave, you can choose how long savasana will last, so you know when your cool-down and seated poses should end. Typically, savasana is three to ten minutes long, depending on the duration of the class.

The wave can be particularly useful if you teach classes of varying duration, as you will probably have to do. Ninety minutes is the traditional length of a yoga class. However, because students' schedules are often so full, more and more studios are offering classes lasting sixty to seventy-five minutes, and corporate yoga classes are usually only forty-five minutes long.

You can use the same class plan more than once in the same week or use it for an entire week, depending on who shows up. Even if a few students attend the repeated classes, you will usually teach them slightly differently, according to your mood and the needs of the students. And you often teach a class better the second or third time through.

Using Themes

One of the biggest questions that comes up in our training classes is whether and how to use themes. Giving a class a specific theme helps you distinguish yoga from mere stretching and creates a richer experience on the mat.

If you keep a journal, on paper or digitally, a great way to generate ideas for themes and anecdotes is to write frequently about how various events in your life relate to yoga and vice versa. If you don't keep a journal, consider carrying a small notebook or creating a digital notepad for this kind of brainstorming.

To use these insights as class themes, you'll need to express them in a way that students can understand and relate to. Even a person who has never heard of the Eight Limbs or the word *Om* should be able to understand what you mean. Ask yourself what makes your insight or theme relevant to everyone in the room.

Telling personal stories can help you relate to your students and get off the teacher's pedestal. But keep them short, especially if the students are sitting in positions that may become uncomfortable and they are anxious to move. Do your best not to focus too much on yourself or your life: not everyone wants to hear a story about your wise and adorable kids in every class. And avoid being self-aggrandizing. It's nice to tell a story in which you learn something, but not one that makes you sound like you're now the most enlightened person on the planet.

Know Why Your Theme Matters

When considering a theme, ask yourself: So what? Why is this relevant and important? Why should anyone care?

It's great if you can link a physical activity theme to a philosophical purpose. For example, when teaching a class with a hip opening emphasis, you might tell your students that opening the hips can be beneficial during difficult times. You might start by saying that hip opening helps you get grounded. But why is getting grounded important? You might explain that being grounded imparts a sense of settled calm to those around you. And why is that important? You might answer that when people around us are settled, they will be living with more kindness and awareness, resulting in more harmony throughout the whole world.

I once took a class in a rural area with an older, experienced teacher who had a strong student base and a very full classroom. At first I really wasn't sure why she was so well respected. However, when she stopped to do an appropriate and succinct demonstration of tree pose for some elderly beginner students in the room, she spoke about how creating strength in the supporting leg would help the students be pillars of strength for their loved ones. Instantly the energy in the room increased, the students' faces lit up, and the remainder of the class was much more captivating and engaging.

Connecting yoga to its highest purpose, even just once per class, can make a huge difference. Here are some categories of themes that can help you do that.

Pulsation-Based Themes

Pulsation (*spanda* in Sanskrit) is reflected everywhere in nature — in the tides coming in and receding, day and night, life and death, light and dark, and so on. In our bodies, we have oppositions like front and back, open and closed, left and right. You can incorporate these ideas into a class theme, encouraging students to find the sweet spot between opposites, which is often a gateway for deeper opening. When you balance the front and back of the body when performing a pose, you usually unfold with more ease. Examples of this type of theme include the following:

- Effort/surrender
- Masculine/feminine
- Courage/contentment
- Intention and desire/letting go

Natural Cycles

Students easily relate to season changes, solstices and equinoxes, and moon cycles, since these are part of our shared experience. Many are starved for nature, so themes like this offer a way to integrate nature into a class and contemplate how we can be inspired by the natural world and its changes.

Yoga Philosophy

If you have a student audience that is open to traditional yoga teachings, you can use lectures or seminars you've attended on yoga philosophy as a great source of themes. The teachings in the texts are infinite: pick something that you and your students can particularly relate to.

Another source of inspiration is the Hindu pantheon of gods and goddesses. Each one, with his or her particular personal attributes and lessons, can provide a theme.

Insights from Your Yoga Practice and Personal Development

Insights and "aha" moments from your own practice and life may be more motivating and exciting to your students than you think — share them! They make wonderful themes. Students enjoy knowing what you are working on and joining in the challenge. For example, you might tell your students, "This month I am focusing on trust and honesty," and invite them to share in that contemplation. Offer a statement of your focus that's catchy and easy to remember, such as "Trust and be true." Some core messages I have heard include the following:

- Gratitude
- Respect
- Letting go of complaining, blaming, justifying, or excuses
- Being open to infinite source and abundance
- Self-compassion
- Living from the heart
- Getting back to the basics

Postural Themes

Postural themes — for example, a focus on the breath, standing poses, shoulders, hips, or endurance — might seem purely physical; however, if you dig deep enough, you'll find they are also meaningful and philosophical. For example, the breath is the link between the physical and the divine. Standing poses engender empowerment and help us cultivate confidence and steadfast remembrance. And the shoulders are connected to the heart center, where we experience vulnerability and love.

The Chakras

The chakras are a rich source of themes, as they represent how we relate to ourselves as well as to the world around us. For example, the root chakra, which is seated in the pelvic floor, has to do with feeling grounded and safe. A whole class can be structured around those qualities while focusing on opening the hips.

Inspiration from the Pinnacle Pose

If your class is structured to build to a pinnacle pose, chances are that this peak pose has a story or an interesting name, or it challenges and opens the body in an enriching and empowering way. For example, ardha chandrasana (half-moon pose), a fairly basic peak pose, has a lot of character! With arms and legs extended, it gives a feeling of flying and freedom, and the supporting leg expresses confidence and stability.

Books, Art, and Movies

Books, art exhibitions, and movies keep you current, inspired, and creative and often supply excellent themes. So do inspiring talks and other cultural events in your community. Students enjoy having their yoga practice come together with something off the mat. After watching *The Wizard of Oz* a few years ago, I was moved by how each character in the story was on their own quest for something they felt they needed in order to be whole. For Dorothy it was finding her way home; for the Scarecrow it was getting a brain; for the Tin Man it was receiving a heart; and for the Lion it was finding courage. Although they started out believing that the Wizard could give them what they sought, they learned that the Wizard was just a little man behind the curtain, and they realized that everything they were seeking was already inside them. Sounds a lot like yoga, right? You can probably imagine the relatable class themes that came out of seeing that movie again!

Celebrations

You can choose a theme related to world or national holidays or a famous person's birthday. Holidays are easy to find using Google, and almost every day is a holiday somewhere in the world! The history of a holiday, as well as the associated traditions, ceremonies, and celebrations, can be of interest. You can also plan a class around a student's birthday, honoring the positive qualities of that person and structuring the practice to cultivate those qualities.

Here in the United States, Valentine's Day and Thanksgiving are two of my favorite holidays. Since Valentine's Day is about love and Thanksgiving is about gratitude, you can't go wrong using them as class themes.

One Valentine's Day, I lined the walkway to the studio with rose petals and lit the room with dozens of soy tea lights. I played schmaltzy, romantic ballads from the seventies and eighties as students entered the studio. I put organic chocolate hearts on everyone's mat during savasana. Realizing that romantic love might be a sensitive or painful theme for some students, I focused the practice on cultivating self-love and allowing relationships to be the "cherry on top" of an already meaningful life.

Chance Inspiration

You never know what might get you and your students fired up. It could be a slogan you saw on a billboard. It could be song lyrics that move you. It could be your children and the deep, funny, and truthful things they say. Be open to inspiration as you go through your day.

Current Events

Current events can affect everyone, and acknowledging them can be very powerful. Whether it is a natural disaster, a community tragedy, or the Olympics, integrating current events into your class themes can deepen the practice.

Life Challenges

Everyone experiences personal tragedy and crisis at some time. You can make these experiences into valuable class themes, showing your students what you learned and who you are now because of them.

I used to think that I couldn't teach while I dealt with personal life challenges. But after trying both subbing out my classes and teaching through the difficult times, I've found that I'm much happier showing up for class and integrating the challenge into my teaching than taking a break.

In the month following the attacks on the World Trade Center in New York City on September 11, 2001, I felt vulnerable and fragile as I attempted to pull myself together to teach. The Wall Street gym where I worked was inaccessible, and most of my students there had been directly affected by the attacks.

When I was able to teach again, I tried to acknowledge the pain everyone felt and uplift them in the face of such madness. It was intense and difficult. At the end of the day, in my apartment, I would fall onto the floor and cry. Yet this experience helped me learn to integrate grieving with teaching. Years later, when I went through a devastating divorce, I didn't miss a class and my teaching felt stronger than ever.

TURNING DIFFICULTY INTO OPPORTUNITY

Yoga is the process of skillfully turning challenges, failures, hurts, and mistakes into opportunities.

Experiencing sadness and pain can offer us insight into how to soothe others in need. The challenges I've lived through fuel my fire to teach others to apply yoga to their lives. I let each of the betrayals, hurts, losses, and crimes light me on fire, then I set every yoga mat in the room on fire (metaphorically speaking, of course!).

If you have lost a loved one, you might dedicate the class to that person's specific virtues and acknowledge how every life leaves blessings for us all. Use the opportunity to explore the idea of living fully now, and guide students to consider the legacy they might want to leave behind.

If you have been betrayed, consider how yoga philosophy and deeper self-awareness could be applied to help you react positively in the face of betrayal. Teach a class focusing on the virtues of truth, friendship, integrity, and making life-affirming choices.

If you are going through a crisis and have a full teaching schedule, teach that the only constant in life is change, and that crisis always brings opportunity. Remember, though, when you're teaching, yoga class is not about you. Take time in private to cry, grieve, and fully feel your experience. Make very sure you have an outlet for anger, disappointment, and hurt so that your students never have to be your therapists. Reach out to peers, counselors, and your teachers for support. When crisis is acute and you are simply too raw to teach, by all means stay home and get your classes covered until you're confident in front of others. Once that happens, even if you are still healing, keep your teaching focused on other things. Otherwise you set your students up to have to take care of you, when during class you should be the one caring for them.

If you do share any part of your crisis, make sure that you're doing it after already having come to some resolution about the crisis, so that you can inspire others to have faith when they are going through difficulty.

GOING THEME-FREE

If you can't focus on a theme and connect it to what you're doing throughout the class, skip it! Classes with no theme can be spacious and allow students to simply practice. I've also seen classes work well where the theme is stated only once at the beginning and not mentioned again, giving students a moment to contemplate a teaching and then letting them apply it in their own way throughout the practice, with no reminder from the teacher. The key with themes is to be aware of what approach you are taking and maintain it.

With the help of your yoga binder, your class plan, and openness to inspiration for class themes, you'll be ready to offer your very best teaching to your students every time you teach a class.

CHAPTER TEN

Teaching a Class

When you deliver a well-thought-out, safe, and inspiring class experience, students will want to return again and again. If your teaching truly inspires them, they may move toward living a lifestyle whose wellspring is yoga, which benefits everyone around them.

Open Up to Receive Divine Direction

If you've had the chance to watch an extremely talented musician perform, it often seems as though some other presence is within them, making their hands play the instrument. The divine pours through them. That power can bring audiences to their feet in a spontaneous standing ovation. We have all experienced the divine to some degree when we are performing, working out, playing sports, dancing, or on the yoga mat: it's the feeling of being "in the zone."

When Michael Jackson passed away, I, like many other people, avidly watched Michael Jackson videos on YouTube. I came across an intimate interview with him. The interviewer asked Jackson, "How do you come up with these things, like where did you come up with that beat in 'Billy Jean'? How is this possible?" Jackson paused and answered, "That's the thing. It did not come from me, that came from up above! Artists have to get out of their own way." This is true for yoga teachers too. When we think too much, we get in our own way and lose the chance to be assisted and inspired by something bigger.

Before you begin teaching, give yourself time to get into a state that allows the divine to pour through you. The students will feel the difference and be moved by the clarity of your offering. Even if your schedule is crowded, try to leave time for a few minutes alone before class to get yourself centered.

WAYS TO BECOME A VESSEL FOR THE DIVINE

Sit with your intention to be a vessel. Meditate on it in whatever way works for you. I close my eyes and concentrate on my breath.

I have found it helpful to do an inversion before class and to chant a beautiful Om.

Focusing on your mission as a teacher, do a ritual or prayer before class, recite mantras in all corners of the room, and give yourself a bit of practice time before class. When I teach pranayama in the beginning of the class, I find it helpful to do the practice with the students when possible.

Parcel It Out

Another incredible talent of Michael Jackson was his ability to tease his audience. He would hold himself back just enough to drive them crazy. He'd restrain his vocals, hold a silent moment for a painfully long time, or restrict his dance movements to a staccato. He wasn't giving them everything they wanted: he was giving them just enough. Girls in the audience would literally pass out from anticipation.

You also see this phenomenon in performances by the best kirtan musicians. Krishna Das, known as the King of Kirtan, is my favorite example. For years he has built his chants slowly and gradually, riding the back of the beat, never letting it play too fast. He'll cast sideways glances at the other musicians and bell players when they start to push the rhythm too quickly. When he finally speeds up, the whole room explodes! People stand up, start dancing, throw their arms in the air, and clap wildly.

You don't need to pull any crazy dance moves in your yoga class or imitate a kirtan singer. Teaching yoga is not a stage performance, but there is something to be said for adopting some of the pacing and restraint of these star artists.

Many teachers make the mistake of saying too much, speaking without ever pausing and giving more information than students can absorb in one class rather than parceling it out in bits and pieces. If you give your students just enough, they will be hungry for more of what you have to offer, both in your group classes and in your other more in-depth offerings. One mistake is trying to cram the content of a three-hour workshop into a sixty-minute class. Students may end up sitting around listening to your opening dharma talk and then watching you demonstrate poses while emphasizing a long list of alignment instructions, when they came to class to move.

Don't be in a rush to impart all your knowledge in one class session. Remember, your classes aren't going anywhere, and hopefully your students aren't either. The biggest compliment I ever received while teaching at a hot flow yoga studio (and I do like to teach alignment-based yoga) was something like, "We sweat and flow, but I always glean some little gem from your classes that helps me go deeper in my poses, Amy." I have a lot of gems to share — far too many to count. You do too. The key is to share those gems just a few at a time so that your students want more.

Presence

Presence is that remarkable ability for a teacher to connect with students in such a way that the students are completely absorbed in what the teacher has to say. Cultivating presence is not simply a matter of innate charisma. It involves conscious effort by the teacher: looking students in the eye, observing them carefully, and getting to know them and their needs. Everyone wants to feel "seen" in this way.

Relating Well to Students

There are a number of simple things you can do (and *not* do!) to make students feel seen, included, welcomed, comfortable, and enthusiastic so that they'll keep coming back to your yoga classes. If you're not sure how well your presentation is going down with students, video recording can be helpful, or you might ask a friend to attend one of your classes and give feedback. Of course, you can also ask your students for feedback, using an anonymous paper or online questionnaire.

Below are some positive habits to cultivate and a few not-so-good ones to eliminate.

Positive Teaching Habits

Here are some pointers for leading a smoothly flowing, rewarding forty-five- to ninety-minute class:

- *Speak succinctly.* Put yourself in the position of your students and try to hear yourself from their perspective. You obviously don't want to tell a long story while your students are holding a difficult pose.
- *Explain why what you are saying is valuable.* It is easy to forget to clearly explain to students why a story, anecdote, myth, or traditional teaching is important, especially when its value is obvious to you. How will this information help them? If you can't come up with an answer, skip the speech!
- *Connect personally with students*, making eye contact with them rather than talking over them.
- *Keep initial centering at the start of class short.* Ideally, wrap it up within three minutes and get your students moving. Five minutes should be the max.
- *Start warm-up with a vinyasa* (one pose per inhale/exhale). In evening classes, most students are coming from work. They have likely sat at a desk all day and now are ready to move. Avoid having these students sit for long periods or talking to them too much right at the beginning. A vinyasa will help them get moving and blow off steam.
- *Come to class prepared.* I can't emphasize this point too strongly. There is nothing worse than a teacher facing a roomful of students and asking, "So, what do you guys want to work on tonight? I didn't have time to prepare."

- *State the class theme* clearly at the start of class and reinforce it one to three times during the class.
- *Pause* to allow students to breathe when in poses.
- *Be spacious in your teaching.* Once you have given your best, most succinct points about alignment and philosophy, allow your students to do their practice, and stick to guiding them in that practice rather than talking more. Some will ask for your assistance; others will cherish a quiet opportunity to execute your instructions and feel the results.
- *Know when a demo is necessary.* When I see that students are struggling to understand my instructions, or I'm teaching a pose they have never seen before, I'll gather them around quickly for a demonstration, either doing the pose myself or asking a student to help me demonstrate. The demo lasts no longer than sixty seconds; otherwise, the students will get antsy. I try to time it to come just after the students have done something fairly strenuous, so that a break is welcome.
- *Attend to every student in the class at least once* with an adjustment or an acknowledgment. I once put up a question on Facebook asking what people wanted more of in yoga class, and the majority responded that they would like more hands-on adjustments. Not everyone wants to be touched, though, so ask first. If they say yes, then get to it. For students who do not want to be touched, offer other forms of acknowledgment, such as making eye contact or addressing them by name. Make a point of giving individual attention to everyone in the room at least once during class. And don't skimp on savasana — give savasana assists as well.

Some of these things will come naturally to you as a teacher, and others may be points you have to work on. It takes a while to reinforce a new habit so that it becomes second nature.

Not-So-Positive Teaching Habits

Here are a few habits that students consistently say they dislike in teachers:

- Talking too much about yourself

- Repeating yourself
- Suggesting that your method of yoga is superior to other methods
- Excessive partner work or demos
- Having "in" jokes with some students
- Departing from the published title or description of the class
- Excessive yoga jargon and clichés

PARTNER WORK

Students who work with people all day or negotiate the needs of family members often do not want to engage in partner work during yoga class. They want their space and a bit of solo time. Some dislike partner work for other reasons, including feeling uncomfortable about touching others or nervous about spotting them. In addition, partner work takes time to explain and arrange and can disrupt the flow of a class. For these reasons, although it may occasionally be useful in sixty- to ninety-minute classes, I think it is best reserved for workshops, retreats, or dedicated partner classes.

In longer-format classes and workshops, partner work can be valuable because it allows everyone to receive hands-on adjustments and spots, enhancing understanding and ability and enabling everyone to advance much faster. To ensure safety, it's important to teach the spot or assist in as much detail as the pose itself. This requires very clear instructions and demonstration, and you'll need to monitor partner work vigilantly to make sure it is being executed properly.

S**T YOGA TEACHERS SAY: STEREOTYPICAL YOGA SPEAK

We asked our Facebook followers to list phrases they thought sounded canned or inauthentic from yoga teachers. The responses included the following:

- "It's all good"
- "Calm your mind"
- "Just be!"
- "Just relax"
- Anything that starts with the word *just!*
- "Let go of your thoughts"
- "Release your monkey mind"
- "Peel away the layers like an onion"
- "Open your heart"

Of course, many of these phrases have become clichés precisely because they contain valuable truths. The way to make them sound less hackneyed is to make them relevant to the lives of your students or give an example of their potency in your own life.

Cultivating New Habits

If any of this feedback from students has made you think there are teaching habits you should change, then make a list of them. Focus on changing them one at a time. It takes one to three weeks of conscious effort to develop a new habit or break an old one. For example, if you tend to talk too much, use the next two weeks to focus on the skill of speaking more economically, with silent pauses to give students the time to experience their poses.

SELL YOUR SUB

When you have to miss a class, let your students know in advance, and praise the teacher you have lined up as a substitute. Although you might legitimately worry that the students will not show up for the sub, not telling them about your absence is unfair to the students and sets them up to be disappointed and dissatisfied when they arrive for class.

One way to strike a positive, community-oriented note is to introduce your sub as a guest teacher rather than a sub. Let the students know that this teacher is a colleague, tell them all the reasons why the teacher is fabulous, and emphasize that you want your students to keep practicing while you're absent. Tell them you want them to stay strong and in "yoga shape" for the things you have planned on your return.

Work with the other teacher to plan what kind of class to teach and maintain continuity in the students' practice. You can then enthusiastically share your guest teacher's class plans and let them know you will be building on those classes when you return. This kind of cooperation and enthusiasm shows that both you and the guest teacher care about the students and about offering quality teaching.

Handling Multiple Ability Levels in Class

Most yoga teachers lead open or multilevel classes. These can be challenging to teach, because if you don't cater to everyone, attendance can suffer.

I've had beginners walk out in horror the minute I asked everyone to come to the wall to attempt to kick into handstand. I've had advanced students popping into full scorpion pose during forearm balance at the wall because they wanted to go deeper. And I've had a student with a truckload of props to modify poses for an acute injury working right next to a yogi with her leg behind her head.

If you're teaching an open-level class, you are implicitly telling students it is safe and appropriate for them to be there. Through trial and much error, I have come up with a number of strategies to make sure I am serving my students well in multilevel classes.

First, give a disclaimer. Clearly state the nature of the class at the start so that you empower the students to take responsibility for their own energy and well-being and to speak up if they need help. Here are some ways to say it:

- "We have multiple levels in class tonight. This is great, because the advanced yogis can help the beginners, and the beginners in the room can help remind the more advanced practitioners about the benefits of slowing down and returning to the basics."
- "There may be poses in class tonight that are outside your physical ability. We have students at different levels, with some who might want the challenge, and some who do not. Please listen to your body, and know that I will always give you a modification if you need one. We have lots of props, so you can still do a version of the pose. It's important to try the modification in order to make progress. So if for any reason I don't see you and you need a modification, please call me over so I can help you!"
- "We've got many different levels in class tonight, so you'll see me giving different options for a few poses. Please pay attention to which option is right for you. Some of us are more flexible in certain poses than in others, and some were born with bodies that do certain things that others do not. It's important not to take any of it personally — just have fun with the option that is right for you, and do it with finesse!"

In your own practice, when you do advanced poses, always keep in mind how you would present them in a mixed-ability class. Think about modifications or alternative variations, and practice them so that you can assist the stiffer students with those variations.

During class, scan the room frequently to assess the ability levels in the class. If you see students struggling, make it a point to smile at them and give them encouragement and stabilizing adjustments without making them feel as if you're singling them out.

By all means, compliment the more advanced students as well, and give them added tips to help them go even deeper, but do it quietly.

If you demonstrate an advanced pose, acknowledge that some students might feel intimidated after seeing it. Then explain and demonstrate the baby steps they can take to eventually get there.

Empower the students with a sequence of poses that make a similar shape to the final, more advanced asana you are building up to. For example, supta padangustasana with the leg out to the side is a similar shape to triangle pose, only you lie on your back. If the students lie on their backs and perform the first pose successfully, they will feel more prepared when you bring them up to do triangle pose standing on their feet.

Be as excited about presenting easier poses as you are about presenting more advanced ones, so that you make it clear that one pose or variation is not better than the other. This way the students will feel good about all the asanas, not just the super-bendy poses!

Timing

Value your students' time. Time is one of the most precious commodities we have. Nothing puts students off more than their time being wasted. They gave up a million other things to be in class with you. Be punctual! Start and end class on time. In addition, pay attention to these areas:

- *Opening talk:* Make it short and to the point. State your theme, and then get your students moving within three to five minutes of starting class.
- *Warm-up:* This should be just long enough to get people prepared for the more challenging poses to come.
- *Inversions:* If you bring a group to the wall and need to work with beginners on fundamentals, the more experienced students may finish quickly and get bored. Give them additional poses or variations to work on so that you can give more time to your beginners.
- *Demos:* An effective demo can be a great use of time, saving you a lot of time explaining things, but keep it brief and clear.
- *Holding poses:* Your students are bound to have varying levels of stamina for holding poses. Whether it's a plank or utkatasana (fierce pose), let students know what benefits they might be getting from the hold so that they stay motivated, and of course give them an alternative if they cannot go the distance.

- *Cool-down:* This needs to be like Goldilocks's bed — not too long, not too short, but just right.
- *Savasana:* As a general rule, allow six to seven minutes for savasana — a minute for getting into the pose, five minutes in it, and a minute to come out. If you are teaching a forty-five- or sixty-minute class, you can make it shorter, but always allow at least three minutes for students to lie still in final relaxation.

CHAPTER ELEVEN

Self-Care

In chapter 9, we talked about the teaching "container," or *dharana*. Throughout this book, we've been discussing all the things that should be in your teaching container: your values and mission statement, good time-management and scheduling, healthy personal and professional relationships, and ways to secure your finances and your ability to contribute as you'd like.

Mission statement · Optimal teaching schedule · Time management · Financial security · Insurance · Contribution (seva) · Healthy relationships · Self-care · Values and vision

These things don't just magically appear in your container: you have to put them there.

We have now looked at every segment shown above except *self-care*. To put it simply, teaching well requires that you are well, and you can truly be well only when you take good care of yourself through healthy habits.

Please don't assume that we are talking about self-care toward the end of the book because it isn't that important. It is.

The sign of a great teacher is one who "walks the talk." It's not enough to preach wellness and healthy habits; you want to live them to such an extent that you are a role model for others. (This doesn't mean you should become so pure in your eating and health habits that no one can relate to you. We are not talking about extremes.)

Imagine taking a class with a teacher who is vibrantly alive, who glows, who obviously attends to his mental, emotional, and physical health. This shows in how he talks, how he listens, how he looks and feels. A person in this state has a twinkle in his eye and is irresistibly appealing; you just want to be around him. In this section we'll look at various ways to nurture yourself so that you can give your best to your students.

Your Own Yoga Practice

Have you ever taken a yoga class when you could just tell that the teacher was not into it? Or have you been that teacher? A passionless teacher can't inspire students. Fortunately, there is a remedy, and that is to get on your own yoga mat and meditation cushion. As the yogini Dana Trixie Flynn puts it, "Just as a concert musician must practice their instrument, a yoga teacher must practice on their mat."

This doesn't mean going to a workshop or retreat only once in a while — though that can be nice — and coming back inspired and enthusiastic. This is about continual refueling. It means getting on your yoga mat consistently, at home, in a class, or at a practice for teachers and advanced students.

This may seem obvious, but the majority of teachers we've polled complain that their single biggest challenge as a teacher is keeping up their own practice. If this is a problem for you, here are some ideas to get you rolling. If you're practicing consistently already, you can skim this section, but you might consider helping to uplift the whole teaching community by organizing group practices that help others stay motivated too.

Establish — and Maintain — Your Home Practice

Having a practice of your own can be not only empowering but often incredibly creative and innovative. If you don't continue to practice regularly in addition to teaching, your only source of inspiration for your teaching is the stale memory of a regular practice. Do whatever it takes to get yourself on your mat five to seven days a week, even if only for a short time. Put on your favorite music first thing in the morning, and get on your mat and just experiment with movement.

Vow to practice at least ten minutes a day, five to seven days a week. By committing to only ten minutes, you avoid putting pressure on yourself, and you're more likely to stick to the resolution. If you start small, you will find yourself craving more time on the mat.

Create a dedicated space in your home for your practice. This will encourage you to practice at home more often. It doesn't have to be anything special — and you certainly don't want to put so much thought into it that the planning process prevents you from rolling out your mat! But when you put just enough energy into a space, it can become magnetic, drawing you onto the mat.

Other tips for practicing consistently and keeping your practice interesting include the following:

- Go straight from your bed to the mat in the morning
- Queue up new music to listen to while practicing
- Attempt a new pose and do a warm-up that gets you there
- Practice someplace new — in a different room, outside, or even in a hot tub
- Lay out your mat in an unavoidable space
- Set a goal for the week, such as a certain number of days on the mat, a certain pose, or more time in a pose
- Keep an asana and meditation journal to stay accountable to yourself
- Write down any inspiring sequences you've done in other teachers' classes or practices, and work on them again

Regularly Practice with Other Teachers

Practicing yoga with other teachers is a vital, synergistic way to build up your yoga practice.

In 2001, I started teaching classes at Laughing Lotus Yoga Center in New York City, founded by the New York yoginis Dana Trixie Flynn and Jasmine Tarkeshi. What I loved about Dana's class was that even after years of teaching yoga, she never seemed to run out of enthusiasm or creativity in her presentations. The excitement was compelling; it made her classes into events you did not want to miss.

When I wondered about the secret to creating this energy, I learned that Dana was on her mat every day, dancing, experimenting, and creating magic.

Dana and I started practicing together weekly at Laughing Lotus, inviting other teachers to join us. I remember those days fondly. The practice was a laboratory for yoga craziness: learning about our bodies and where we needed to develop strength, where we needed to open up, experimenting with zany poses, making up new ones, figuring out how best to get into advanced poses, and more. We did timings and repetitions, played ridiculous music, and laughed.

That spirit of creativity and togetherness led to some of the biggest breakthroughs in my yoga practice. When I moved to Colorado in 2004 and discovered a teachers' practice called "The Tigress," I felt at home again.

If there's nothing similar in your area, consider organizing your own informal practice for teachers and advanced practitioners. It's a terrific way to advance your practice and keep yoga exciting.

Here are some tips for organizing a teachers' practice:

- Pick a time based on the availability of the teachers in your area, either by doing a survey or doing some online research on teachers' schedules.
- Find a yoga studio to host the practice during off hours, preferably as a community service to the local teachers.
- When you have settled on a location and meeting time, send an email invitation to all the teachers.
- Start a group or create an event page for the practice on social media. Post pictures and even videos to get people inspired. Be consistent and show up yourself. Repeat: *Be consistent and show up yourself!*
- Send out a reminder email the day before each practice, and let the group know what cool things might be occurring at the practice, such as holiday or birthday celebrations, or a specific pose the practice will build to.
- Celebrate birthdays, holidays, and milestones, and regularly dedicate your practices to students in the community and anyone in need.
- Choose an experienced teacher to lead the practice (it might be you), or have all the teachers take turns as leader.

Another way to keep your own practice fresh is to attend other teachers' classes and workshops in your community. This not only benefits your yoga practice but also increases your visibility. Chances are that your attendance at your peers' classes will be reciprocated. When they come to your classes, you can mention their presence to your students and compliment their teaching, showing a spirit of camaraderie, collaboration, and generosity in the studio.

Mental and Emotional Health

Keeping your mind sharp and clear is key to great teaching. Unresolved conflicts with people you love or work with can sap your energy and make you preoccupied and less present in the classroom.

If you're dealing with unresolved conflicts with family, friends, colleagues, or others, can you clear the air? How about your relationship to your significant other? Are you tending to your partner's needs and expressing your own?

One way to tend to your emotional health and find paths out of conflict is to keep a journal where you can blow off steam or vent. Another is to express yourself through art. If you have a creative pastime that you've been neglecting, maybe now is the time to take it up again.

Here are some other options to consider to lift your spirits:

- *Get a massage or bodywork.* After a massage, I feel like I can do anything! Being touched changes my whole mood and outlook on life and makes me want to give back to others.
- *Have a vacation planned.* Knowing that there is a light at the end of the work tunnel can give you a lot more energy.
- *Be more social.* Schedule time to be enriched by the company of friends. If you're in a relationship, plan get-togethers with other friends to enjoy the benefits of community.

Your Physical Appearance and Well-Being

This may seem superficial, but attending to your appearance can make a huge difference to your sense of well-being and self-esteem. A yoga teacher who projects vibrant energy and radiance makes a great role model for health and wellness. Looking and feeling good instantly gives you more professionalism and presence.

Consider these areas:

- *Exercise:* Are you getting ample cardiovascular exercise besides yoga? Moving and getting your heart rate up is invigorating. I recently started learning a new sport, skate skiing. It is very aerobic

and works the whole body. It leaves me feeling like an Ironwoman, full of life and uplifted from the sun's reflection on the snow.
- *Diet:* Are you eating clean, nourishing meals?
- *Skin care:* Could your skin glow more? Problem skin may be a sign of a nutritional or sleep deficiency.
- *Hair:* When your hair is nicely styled and cut regularly, you'll come across as more professional.
- *Hygiene:* When you arrive for class looking and feeling fresh, you'll project a more energetic and healthy image. Bring deodorant in your bag in case you have a stinky moment.
- *Feet:* Pedicures are a perfect treat for yoga teachers, since we are barefoot so much of the time, and students do look at our feet.

Taking care of yourself and your appearance can be expensive, but it's an investment in your career and teaching. When you are healthy, vibrant, and looking and feeling good, opportunities come your way, and your classes become more energized.

Organization

As we talk about organizing your teaching, I can't resist adding a note about organizing the rest of your life. Obviously, that's a big subject, but I have seen remarkable results from tackling aspects of it.

Take some time to organize your possessions. If you're sitting in a cluttered office space, it's likely you'll have less energy, lack creativity, and have poor self-esteem. A messy closet can cause you to spend fifteen minutes looking for a misplaced yoga top when you could have been on your mat practicing — or planning a class.

When you declutter your home, you release natural endorphins that give you a surge of pleasure and energy. When my mother inherited my grandmother's possessions, I recommended that she hire a professional organizer to help declutter the house. My mom had done yoga sporadically for years but was not what I'd call a yogini. And yet when she saw what she and the organizer had done in her office, she reported having what I could only call a *kundalini* experience. Decluttering sent a liberating energy through her spine and out the crown of her head, one that gave her a lasting sense of possibility and potential.

    I experienced these benefits for myself when my mom gifted me my own session with a professional organizer. I am still using the filing system we set up, I know how and when to purge closets and rooms, and I can keep, toss, and organize much more efficiently. Though I use these systems predominantly in my personal life, they extend into my professional life as well.

CONCLUSION

Light Up the World

To be a yoga teacher is to embody what it means to have well-being in life, and in turn to impart that understanding to others. Teaching yoga is a sacred calling for many. Indeed, it is one of the most rewarding professions out there — not many others can say that it's their job to make people feel good!

Much of this book has been about how to skillfully serve, inspire, and assist yoga students. Yet perhaps the most rewarding part of this profession is the one that centers on ourselves. Being a yoga teacher grants each of us the opportunity to be a lifelong student and create a more meaningful life for ourselves. It's a career that has self-care, self-inquiry, and self-discovery built right into the job description. The perks are seemingly endless: enhanced self-awareness, learning, community, and a personal yoga practice that supports our body, heart, and mind for years to come.

Ironically, the more we "selfishly" benefit from yoga and a career in yoga, the more we excel in our teaching and as a result mobilize our students to shift their own lives for the better. Ultimately, we study yoga and train in yoga to know ourselves more deeply, and when we radiate that self-awareness is when we shine brightest as teachers. One thing I know for sure is that great yoga teachers make the world a more peaceful, intelligent, and conscious place to be.

Refer to these pages for inspiration often. Take action on the ideas that resonate most. Keep studying the vast infinitude that is yoga philosophy, asana, pranayama, and meditation. Study anatomy and biomechanics. And be a lifelong student of business and marketing so that your yoga has the proper vehicle to get out into the world!

Trust yourself and your own authentic seat as the teacher. Carve out and claim the time to care for yourself, do your practice, and kindle your own fire. Then watch how your enthusiasm and energy can light up another's life. This is how we help wake up the world.

Index

Page references in italic type indicate illustrations.

abdominals/core work, 142
accountants, 66, 122
acquiring students, 62–63
Advaita Vedanta, 8
advertising in wellness publications, 93
Affordable Health Care Act ("Obamacare"), 124
The Alchemical Body (White), 11
apex pose, 140, 142
appearance, physical, 173–74
ardha chandrasana (half-moon pose), 147
arm balances, 142
art as a source of themes, 148
asana, 15
athletes, 61
auchitya (filled with appropriateness), 22

bank accounts, 122–23
beauty, 26
Beck, Martha, 23–24
beginner classes, 44–46, 57–58, 70–71
Bitly.com, 108
bookkeepers, 66, 122
books as a source of themes, 148
brand, 84–86
breath, 147
Brooks, Douglas, 84
Buffer, 109
building your business, 65–80; business plan, 35, 65–66; money professionals, 66; opening your own studio, 78–80; payment models, 74; quitting your day job, 71–72; résumé, 66–67; in rural areas, 70–71; scheduling, optimal, 74–78; student base, 74; sustainable teaching, 72–78; teaching opportunities, 67–70
Bunch, Jim, 32

business basics, 43–64; beginner classes, 44–46, 57–58; conferences, 51; continuing education, 57–58; endorsements, 52, 107; etiquette for new students, 45; festivals, 51; finances, 55–56; gift certificates, 59; group classes, 47, 57, 59; partnerships, 52; private lessons, 43, 47–48, 57, 59; product sales, 51–52; retreats, 43, 50, 58; schools, teaching in, 54–55; specialty classes, 46, 58; student base, building, 59–64; teacher training, 48–50; teaching schedule, balanced, 56–59; workplaces, teaching in, 53–54; workshops, 43, 48, 58. *See also* building your business

business cards, 93

business entity, creating, 122

business plan, 35, 65–66

"California Yoga Teachers Association Code of Conduct" (Lasater), 20

Canfield, Jack, 32

celebration-based themes, 148–49

centering, 141, 157

chakras, 147

chanting, 154–55

charisma, 23–24

charitable contributions, 125–26

class preparation, 129–52; anecdotes, 144; benefits of, 129, 137; binder for teaching, 130–36; class plans, 132–33; cues/instructions for poses, 133–34; disadvantages of, 137; how much to plan, 136–37; importance of, 158; inspirational message, 132; for mini-vinyasa flows, 135; music, 141; packing list (items needed for class), 130; personal challenges, incorporating into teaching, 150; quotations, 135; rehearsing what you'll teach, 131; sequencing class elements, 141–43; student/client notes, 135; template for, *138–39*, 138–43; themes, 132, 140, 143–51; traditional length of class, 143; verbs used in yoga, 136

class size, 76–77

class teaching, 153–65; acknowledgment of students, 158; centering, 157; cooling down, 165; demos, 158, 164; divine direction, 153–54; holding poses, 165; imparting just enough knowledge, 154–56; individual attention to students, 158; inversions, 164; multiple ability levels in class, 162–64; opening talk, 164; partner work, 159–60; preparation for, 158 (*see also* class preparation); presence, 156; relating well to students, 156; savasana, 158, 165; stereotypical yoga speak, 160; substitutes during your absence, 161; teaching habits, cultivating new, 161; teaching habits, negative, 159; teaching habits, positive, 157–59; themes, 158; timing, 164–65; warming up, 157, 164

clutter, 174–75

colleagues, relationship with, 118–20

community, 99

competition, 85

conferences, 51, 93–94

conflict, 172–73

consumerism, 11

continuing education/practice, 14, 57–58, 168–69

cooling down, 142, 165

core/abdominals work, 142

core values, 29–33, 131

corporate yoga, 53–54

counterposes, 142

Coursera.com, 100
crises, working through, 149–51
current events, 149
cycles in nature, 145–46

dakshina (sacred compensation or sacrifice), 9
Das, Krishna, 117, 155
dharana (container), 129, 137, 167, *167*
diet, 174
the divine, relationship with, 116
divine direction, 153–54

ego, 35
email, 91, 96
emotional health, 172–73
endorsements, 52, 107
ethical issues: code of ethics, 19; money, 6–11, 81; responsibility, 22–23; *yamas* and *niyamas*, 20–22, 132
etiquette for new students, 45
exemplary teachers, 17, 19–24
exercise, 173–74
eye contact, 157

Facebook, 70, 92, 96–97, 101–5
family/friends, relationship with, 116–17
fashion sense, 27–28
feedback, 156
festivals, 51
finances. *See* money
flexibility, physical, 27
flyers, marketing via, 91
Flynn, Dana Trixie, 168, 170–71
foot care, 174
Franklin, Benjamin, 33

gender of teachers, 27
gift certificates, 59
grieving, 150–51
groundedness, importance of, 144
group classes, 47, 57, 59, 68–69
guest teaching, 67–68

hair, 174
health insurance, 123–24
Hindu gods and goddesses, 146
hip opening, 144, 147

holiday-based themes, 148–49
home practice, 169–70
Hootsuite, 109
Horan, Jim: *The One Page Business Plan*, 65
humility, 23
hygiene, 174

inhaling/exhaling, cues for, 133
insights that motivate, 146–47
inspiration, being open to, 149
Instagram, 92, 97, 100–101, 105–7
insurance, 123–25
inversions, 142, 164
investment account, 123
Iyengar, B. K. S., 28

Jackson, Michael, 153–55
Jois, Pattabhi, 28

karma, 20–21, 23
kirtan, 117, 155

Lasater, Judith Hanson: "California Yoga Teachers Association Code of Conduct," 20
Laughing Lotus Yoga Center (New York City), 170–71
Lee, Cyndi, xi
liability insurance/release forms, 124–25
life challenges, 149–51
lifestyle business, 4
lighting up the world, 177–78
lila (divine play), 21–23
LinkedIn, 66, 102
loyalty building, 64, 117

Madonna, xii
marketing, 81–94; advertising, 93; assets/goals, 82, 84–85; brand, 84–86; business cards, 93; data analysis, 88–89; via email, 96; five Ps of, 89–90; ideal students, identifying, 37–39, 86–88; marketing funnel, *83*, 83–84; message, 82; offerings, 82–83, 89; planning, 56, 90–92; self-assessment of, 28; via social media, 28, 97 (*see also* social media); spreading the word, 82–83; target market, 86–89; traditional, 93–94
massage, 173
meditation, 10, 142, 154
mental health, 172–73
microblogging, 101
Millennials, 96
mini-vinyasa flows, 135
mission statement, 33, 35–36, 131

money: annual income, 55–56; as aspect of successful teachers, 27; hiring professionals, 66, 122; managing, 121–26; and quitting your day job, 71–72; and teaching, 6–11, 13, 81
motivational insights, 146–47
movies as a source of themes, 148
multilevel classes, 162–64

natural cycles, 145–46
networking, in-person, 94
newsletters, 93
new students, etiquette for, 45
"90 Minutes to Change the World," xiv, 11, 89
90 Monkeys, xiii–xiv, 31, 45

"Obamacare" (Affordable Health Care Act), 124
The One Page Business Plan (Horan), 65
oneself, relationship with, 116
open-level classes, 162–64
organizing your life/possessions, 174–75
The Origins of Yoga and Tantra (Samuel), 11

parents, new, 60–61
partnerships, 52
partner work in class, 159–60
Patanjali, 8, 10, 20–21
paying yourself first, 122
pedicures, 174
philosophy of yoga, 146
physical appearance, 173–74
physical prowess, 27
pinnacle pose, 140, 142
Pinterest, 110
poses: ardha chandrasana (half-moon pose), 147; counterposes, 142; cues/instructions for, 133–34; holding, 165; in multilevel classes, 162–63; pausing for breathing, 158; pinnacle, 140, 142, 147; pulsation-based, 145; seated, 142; standing, 141–42, 147; supta padangustasana, 164; twist (ardha matsyendrasana), 134
position of product, 90
postcards, marketing via, 91
postural themes, 147
prakriti, 10, 10–11
pranayama, 154
presence, 156
price, 90
private lessons, 43, 47–48, 57, 59
products/services, 51–52, 89
professionalism, 68–69
professional relationships, 27, 115–20
promotion, 90–91. *See also* marketing

pulsation (*spanda*), 145
purusha, *10*, 10–11

Qualman, Erik: *Socialnomics*, 96–97
questionnaires, 38, 62, 88, 156
quotations, 135

Ramayana, xiv
referrals, 93
Registered Yoga Teacher, 67
responsibility, 22–23
résumés, 66–67
retaining students, 63–64
retreats, 43, 50, 58

Samuel, Geoffrey: *The Origins of Yoga and Tantra*, 11
savasana (final relaxation), 143, 158, 165
savings account, 123
scheduling, optimal, 74–78
schools, teaching in, 54–55
seated poses, 142
self-assessment/-presentation, 17–39; background, 28; beauty, 26; being true to yourself, 26; charisma, 23–24; connection with well-known teachers, 28–29; core values, 29–33; ethical principles, 20–23; the exemplary teacher, 17, 19–24; fashion sense, 27–28; financial security, 27; gender, 27; ideal students, identifying, 37–39; improvement, identifying areas for, 29; marketing acumen, 28; mission statement, 33, 35–36; the nonexemplary teacher, 24–25; physical prowess, 27; professional connections, 27; responsibility, 22–23; the skilled teacher, 17–18; the successful teacher, 17, 25–29; timing of career, 27; understanding why you teach, 33–35; the unskilled teacher, 19; yoga pedigree, 28–29
self-awareness, 177–78
self-care, 116, 167–75
seva (service), 125–26
skilled teachers, 17–18
skin care, 174
Smith, Taro, xiii
Snapchat, 110
social media, 52, 70, 92–93, 95–113; basics of, 100–102; benefits of, 95–97; community on, 99; connections on, 99; content shared on, 98–99, 101; curating your content on, 99–101, 104; email, 96; Facebook, 96–97, 101–5; fame via, 106–7; fear of, 97–98; haters on, 111–12; Instagram, 97, 100–101, 105–7; LinkedIn, 102; marketing via, 28, 97; personal info on (transparency), 110–13, *111*; Twitter, 97, 107–10
Socialnomics (Qualman), 96–97
social time, 173
spiritual bypassing, 22
spiritual enlightenment, 8
staff, relationship with, 118–20
standing poses, 141–42

Stein, Ben, 116
Sting, xii
student base, building, 59–64
student/client notes, 135
studio, attending functions at, 118–19
studio, opening your own, 78–80
substitute teaching, 67–68, 161
successful teachers, 17, 25–29
succinct teaching, 157
sun salutation, 133
supta padangustasana, 164
survivor stories, 28
sustainable teaching, 72–78

Tantra, 11
Tarkeshi, Jasmine, 170
teacher-student relationship: connecting with students, 156–57; ethics in, 20–22; maintaining, 117
teacher training, 48–50
teaching a class. *See* class teaching
teaching schedule, balanced, 56–59
teaching today, 3–15, 4; challenges of, 6; free classes, 7–8; good news about, 4–6; and money, 6–11, 13, 81; scope of, 14–15; training hours/programs, 13–14; vicious cycle of yoga teaching, 11–13
timing of career, 27
twist pose, cues for, 134
Twitter, 92, 97, 107–10

Uno (prize-winning beagle), 23–24
URL links, 108

vacations, 173
Valentine's Day, 148–49
value propositions, 60–62
values, core, 29–33, 131
verbs used in yoga, 136
vicious cycle of yoga teaching, 11–13
vinyasa yoga, 133, 135, 157

warming up, 141–42, 157, 164
website, marketing via, 91
White, David G.: *The Alchemical Body*, 11
The Wizard of Oz as a source of themes, 148
word-of-mouth sharing, 96. *See also* social media
workplaces, teaching in, 53–54
workshops, 43, 48, 58

yamas and *niyamas*, 20–22, 132

yoga: benefits of, 3, 5; benefits of teaching, 177–78; commercialization of, 6–7; and environmental/social issues, 5; growth/popularity of, xii, 4–6; home practice, 169–70; number of students, 4; philosophy of, 146; schools/traditions of, 8, 10–11; spending on, 4, 8; Tantric schools of, 11; teachers' practice, 170–72; vinyasa, 133, 135, 157

Yoga Alliance, 4, 13–14, 67

"Yoga in America" study, 4–5, 39

Yoga Journal, 4, 39, 125

Yoga Journal Teachers Plus, 125

Yoga Sutras of Patanjali, 10, 20–21

yoga teachers, perceptions of, xii. *See also* teaching today

www.ingramcontent.com/pod-product-compliance
Lightning Source LLC
Chambersburg PA
CBHW081158020426
42333CB00020B/2546